Healing with medicinal plants

MW01032349

Healing with Medicinal Plants
basis for their use - second edition

Written by:
Cecilia Garcia, Chumash Healer and Spiritual Leader. Ensenada, Mexico.
and
James David Adams, Jr., Associate Professor, University of Southern California, School of Pharmacy, Los Angeles, CA 90089. Tel: (323) 442-1362. Email: jadams@usc.edu.

Published by:
Abedus Press
PO Box 8018
La Crescenta, CA 91224-0018

ISBN - 0-9763091-3-0
First printing 2005

Library of Congress Control Number: 2004115239 first edition
Garcia, Cecilia and Adams, James David.
Healing with Medicinal Plants of the West – cultural and scientific basis for their use - second ed.
Includes bibliographical references (p.) and index.
ISBN 0-9763091-3-0 second edition

Contents

About the Authors

Cecilia Garcia is a Chumash Healer. She learned Chumash healing from her maternal and paternal Grandparents who were all Chumash Healers. She has practiced her healing arts on many people over the years. Cecilia practices the Chumash religion, which is integral to Chumash healing. She has a generous spirit and has openly shared her knowledge in this book.

James David Adams, Jr. is an Associate Professor of Molecular Pharmacology and Toxicology at the University of Southern California. He got his PhD in 1981 at UC San Francisco in Comparative Pharmacology and Toxicology. He has been involved in learning Chumash healing since 1998. All plant photographs are by Jim Adams.

Forward – By Ted Garcia (2005), Wot (Chief) of the San Fernando Valley Chumash people March, 2009

In the late 1950's my Grandmother brought her brothers, sisters and members of the family together. She was Chumash and part Tongva. She was a spokesperson for the family, and the one who taught us to respect others. When she became elderly and not in good health, my Father's first cousin, Charlie Cook, was named our Chief and became the spokesman for our family.

About ten years ago, I got back into my culture. I became a stone carver. I carve soapstone in the Chumash way. I also learned to bless people with white sage and a feather fan. My Cousin taught me how to bless, smudge white sage and use the fan. Soon my family, especially my wife, asked me to bless our family. Now, I bless people at family gatherings and social events.

Blessing is all about helping the person being blessed to find positive energy. In a social setting, it is important to have positive energy. A person with negative energy attracts more negativity. Soon that person may carry a huge load of negativity. We all run across negative people and negative situations. That negativity should be cleansed away before entering into a family setting or social event.

Blessing with white sage smoke cleanses and helps people find a positive attitude. It is a symbolic washing. The person being blessed symbolically draws the smoke to the head, to wash the hair and face, then draws the smoke to the heart, to cleanse the heart and spirit. When I bless, I start from the top of the head and go to the feet. Then I go behind from the top of the head to the feet. I ask the person being blessed to raise each foot so I can smudge the bottoms of the feet. This cleanses the whole body. I use my fan to fan away negative energy the person may have.

I pray for the person I am smudging. If a man is in poor health, I pray that his health will be brought back to him. If a woman is in a bad situation, I pray that she will get through it. Basically, what I do is ask the Creator to let the person not bring harm to others and to let no harm come to the person. I also ask that the person should make the right decisions and go on the right path. I also ask the person being blessed to pray for something personally special. The man who taught my Cousin said "I always pray for world peace." I think there is very great

4

power in prayers to the Creator. Prayers are positive, so that positive energy comes back to the one praying. Prayers are a process of looking for something positive. Many of these prayers have been answered.

Blessing my family is very important to me, because without them, I am nothing. I measure wealth by what I have in my family, not by money. I tell other people that having a steady job and being able to provide for the family is very important.

When I am blessing, I really concentrate on what I say before I say anything. I know that what I say can make an impact on people. Any impact I have, I want to be good and positive. These blessings at social events can help us all come together and heal the separations between us, not just the Native Community. I think it is important for all cultures to come together, because first and foremost we are all human beings.

Acknowledgements –
        Many people have taught the authors about plants, photography and Indian culture. Chumash people we want to thank are Frank Lemos, Denice Garcia, Paul Varela, Ruth Frazee, David Franks and David Dominguez. Other Indian people we thank are Jan Cleary, Julia Bogany (Tongva), Jorge Hernandez (Viejas) and Phil Johnson (Miwok). Forest Rangers and Park Biologists have helped us learn about and locate plants including Darrell R. Wanner, Larry R. Saslaw, David Clendenen, Michael C. Long, Scott D. White, Paul Seiley, Dana York, Ken Low, David Numer, Tony Smock and Tom Chester. Several botanic gardens have been very useful to the authors especially Rancho Santa Ana Botanic Garden (Michael Wall), the University of California Riverside Botanic Garden, the Living Desert and Santa Barbara Botanic Garden (Betsy Collins). We are especially grateful to Dr. Michael Wall for checking all of the plant identifications in the book. Barbara J. Collins of the California Lutheran College has been very helpful in teaching, through her website, the authors about plant identification. Some nurseries have been very helpful including the Tree of Life Nursery in San Juan Capistrano and the Theodore Payne Foundation in Sunland. The authors are grateful to Joan DeFato of the Arboretum of Los Angeles County for providing useful notes on medicinal plants. We also would like to thank John R. Johnson and Jan Timbrook of the Santa Barbara Museum of Natural History for several useful email discussions and for sending useful publications. Dr. Lowell Bean has provided the authors with valuable information about Cahuilla plants and culture. Richard Applegate of Santa Rosa Junior College, provided the pronunciations of Chumash words. All Chumash words are in the Ventura Chumash dialect, because that is the area Cecilia Garcia's ancestors came from. Jim Adams has added the pronunciation of the glottal stops. He is an expert in the pronunciation of glottal stops since he speaks Cantonese, a language that has many glottal stops. The authors are grateful to Philip Bedel of the Santa Monica Mountains National Recreation Area for teaching us about plant photography. Robert Roberts created the photograph of Pogonomyrmex californicus. Robert Roberts and Chris Schweska of the University of Southern California, School of Pharmacy were very helpful with photographic advice and assistance.

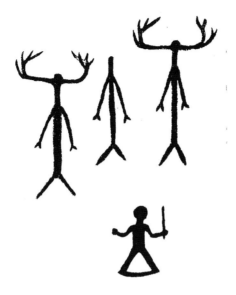

The Deer Dance occurs in December to ensure that deer will always be available. The swordfish, below, ensures that food will be available in the winter. Drawings are by Jim Adams.

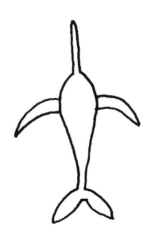

Warning-Disclaimer

This book was written to be used as a self help manual for people interested in learning healing and using western plants in this healing process. The recommendations for use of the plants are solely the authors' opinions and may not be valid for all people. Each person is different and may have a different response to any given plant. The recommendations are general guidelines that are designed to provide a safe approach for the use of the plants in most people. Any plant is toxic at a high enough dose. There may be unknown adverse effects of the plants or insects that are not reported and not known to the authors. Any plant preparation can cause allergic reactions, even anaphyllaxis, if used too frequently. The authors do not accept any responsibility of any kind for any possible adverse affects of any plant or insect preparation in any person at any time.

Please be aware that whenever you use a plant in healing or for nourishment, you do so at your own risk. You use this book at your own risk. You must accept the responsibility for proper identification and use of each plant. You must accept the responsibility to use the proper dose of each plant. Please be aware that some plant preparations may have dangerous interactions with drugs or other plant preparations. You are responsible for accepting the possible dangers of these interactions, known or unknown. You are responsible for properly cultivating these plants for your own use. You may not collect plants in the wild without the proper permit.

All doses and preparations given in this book are approximate. You should use the dose and amount of plant material that feels correct to you. Be aware that moderation and mild preparations are normal among the Chumash people. Teas and other preparations are normally very mild.

The Healing Way
In the old days, it was believed that some people were born with the gift of healing. This was a hereditary gift that tended to be present in some families, but not others. The knowledge of how to use this gift was usually passed from the Grandparents to the Grandchildren. Of course, everyone had knowledge of how to use certain plants to heal themselves and their families. But the medicine people had an extra ability to heal. The gift to heal was frequently recognized at a young age. The future Healer was taken under the guidance of a family member, who was already a Healer. Among some California Indian groups, such as the Chumash and Yokuts, the best Healers were educated at schools of medicine to learn about healing and how to use plants. The most well known school of medicine was in the Cuddy Valley, called 'Antap in Chumash (pronounced gontop), near Mount Pinos. The medical school education lasted for a year. However, learning about healing was a life long process. Each Healer knew that the learning process was not complete at the end of the medical school education. After this education, the young Healer became an apprentice to a recognized Healer. The apprenticeship lasted for seven years, until the apprentice had developed the proper maturity to use the healing gift wisely. The gift to heal was understood to be a sacred gift.

Prayer was an essential part of healing. Prayers were used when medicinal plants were harvested. Prayers were recited when people were treated with these plants. God was involved in the healing process, just as God should be involved in healing today. Most medicine people lived on song and prayer, although they were well paid for their healing. Unfortunately, modern medicine treats the body and neglects the spirit. In the old days, the spirit was treated first, then the body. The body was understood to be just a carrier for the spirit. Most disease was believed to start with the spirit, such as when the spirit decided to become sick, or when the spirit forgot how to be well.

Dreaming was an essential part of wellness. Pleasant dreams can cure the spirit or maintain the wellness of the spirit. Dreaming can help the spirit remember how to be happy, and how to be well. Unpleasant dreams may damage the spirit leading to disease. Mugwort had an important role in helping to produce pleasant dreams.

In the old days, medicine people had senses of humor.

9

When a person was sick from having a too difficult or complex life, the medicine people tried to help the sick person laugh at the problems. The medicine people did not want the sick person to fret about the illness, because this would prevent healing. The medicine people helped the sick person remember how to be well.

"When you are sick, I will tell you how silly you are. You're not allowing yourself to be well. You're taking on the world's misery. You have lost your sense of self. You're like a three year old whining. You need my love. You need my attention. And I'm going to give it to you. I'm going to hand you things to do, so that you will get over yourself and fit back as a useful member of society." Cecilia Garcia (Chumash)

Plants are blessings from God. The knowledge of how to use the plants is also a gift from God. When a Healer needs a plant to treat an unfamiliar disease, the Healer goes out among the plants until she feels drawn to a certain plant. The Healer prays and spends up to four days near the plant, even sleeping near the plant. God directs the Healer in the use of the plant to treat the disease. This is how many unfamiliar diseases came to be treated by California Indians, such as flu, dysentery, measles and malaria.

Medicine people can activate plants to make them work for any condition. That is why there are so many secondary uses for some plants. Someone with the gift of healing can use any plant that is available to treat a sick person. This is very convenient when the plant of first choice is not available. In addition, Healers can successfully treat certain conditions with prayer and plants, even when other people cannot.

"I have a love for this. I am a woman. I have the purity and simplicity of blind faith that creates my ability to comfort. It is my sincerity that I believe so strongly, that creates my ability to heal." Cecilia Garcia (Chumash)

An essential part of health in the old days was prevention of sickness. This meant maintaining good spiritual health and doing hard work. Everyone was expected to be a productive member of society and to work hard every day for the village. Each person knew their function in society, knew that their part was essential and did not want to miss a day of work. Of course, working for the village has two benefits, it keeps each person physically fit and makes each person feel needed. This can maintain mental and physical health. In the old days, few people were very overweight because they worked hard every day.

It is real important that the plants are in your life, that you are taking white sage. Put a leaf of white sage in your coffee. Put a leaf of white sage in the water you drink. It is important to get the medicine in you. The medicinal plants and the knowledge of their use should be part of our lives and should be shared. God gave these plants to the California Indians to use and to share with everyone. They are not for the greedy.

Plants must be collected properly, such as from your own garden. It is not legal to collect plants in most parks, forests or other public land, without a permit. Permits can be obtained from the rangers or park officials in many areas. When plants are collected with a permit, be sure to not collect more than ten percent of the plant material. For instance, take no more than ten leaves for every one hundred leaves from a bush of white sage. This will help the plant grow back stronger and ensure more plant material in the future. For small plants, do not collect more than ten percent of the plants in the area. If there are thirty of the plants in the area, take no more than three of them. This will ensure that the plants can propogate, so there will be more in the future.

The gift to heal can be lost. It can be lost by hoarding it and not sharing it. It can be lost by crossing the lines of morality as judged by society. Moral purity is essential to a medicine person. When society judges that a Healer is no longer morally pure, that person has lost the ability to heal. The Healer is just a tool of God. The Healer must not forget this, and must not aggrandize himself, or the gift will be lost. The gift to heal can also be lost by losing faith. The gift comes from God. The Healer must have an unshakable faith.

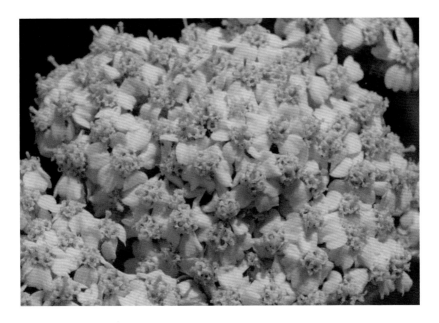

Scientific name – Achillea millefolium
Common name – Yarrow

Identification – This plant is usually about two feet tall. The leaves are alternate and very finely pinnately divided. The flowers form in large heads of many small, white flowers. The flowers can also be pink or yellow. The ligules are about an eighth of an inch long (1).

Characteristics – Yarrow usually has a pleasant smell. It is found in canyons and mountain areas, including Mount Pinos, up to nearly 10,000 feet in elevation.

Distribution – This plant grows throughout the Pacific States and is a common plant (2). Very similar and chemically related species occur in North America, Europe and Asia (3).

Primary uses – Yarrow was used as a pain reliever in tooth ache, arthritis, head ache and colds (4).

"We take our medicine softly and neutrally. Sucking on a yarrow leaf gives the proper dose that the body can absorb. Suck on it until it loses its flavor." Cecilia Garcia (Chumash)

Secondary uses – This plant was used as a poultice for wounds to control swelling and hemorrhaging. Some Indians treated broken bones by holding the area over steaming yarrow leaves, then binding the area with steamed buckskin strips (4).

Active compounds – Achillea species contain many active compounds, including some anti-inflammatory compounds such as a germacrane, stigmasterol, beta-sitosterol, rupicolin B and a matricarin derivative (3). These compounds should help relieve pain and swelling.

Recommendations – Yarrow is a widely used plant, especially used as a tea. However, the tea probably does not contain some of the anti-inflammatory compounds found in the plant, that are not very water soluble. Yarrow tea is used in Europe for mild cramps in the guts. It is probably safe and better to use the leaves of yarrow for pain relief. Sucking on two leaves may help against pain. It is probably safe to apply a poultice of yarrow leaves to a swollen area. Discontinue use if a rash forms. Hemorrhage should be treated by applying direct pressure to the bleeding area, not by making a yarrow poultice. Broken bones should never be bound with steamed strips of buckskin. Upon drying the buckskin may become so tight that blood flow may be restricted. This may result in loss of the affected arm or leg. A broken bone should be treated by a health care provider.

Healing with medicinal plants by Garcia and Adams

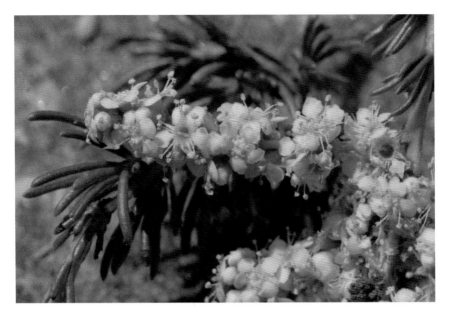

Scientific name – Adenostoma fasciculatum
Common name – Chamise

Identification – Chamise grows as a bush up to 10 feet tall, but is
usually less than 6 feet tall. The bark is gray-brown. The leaves
are less than half an inch long, needle shaped and more abundant
than red shank leaves (1). Small, white flowers form as bracts in
the Spring.

Characteristics – Chamise is a perennial and grows abundantly in
chaparral below about 4,000 feet. It is usually the most common
plant in the chaparral. Chamise and red shank can sometimes be
found growing near each other. However, chamise usually grows
at lower elevations than red shank (1). Chamise leaves have very
little smell or flavor.

Distribution – Chamise is common throughout Baja California,
Southern and Central California and is found in part of Northern
California (1).

Primary uses – An infusion of chamise bark or a salve made from
twigs was used for skin infections and sores. The leaves were

14

used as a tea for stomach ulcers, colds and respiratory problems (4).

Secondary uses – The tips of arrow shafts were commonly chamise. The coals from chamise were good for roasting food.

Active compounds – Adenostoma fasciculatum and A. sparsifolium contain flavonoids such as kaempferol, quercetin and isorhamnetin (5). Phenolic acids are also present (5).

Recommendation – Chamise is probably safe to use for sores, colds and flus. It can probably be used along with standard therapy for ulcers, provided that your Pharmacist is consulted about this. Skin infections and respiratory tract infections should be treated with antibiotics.

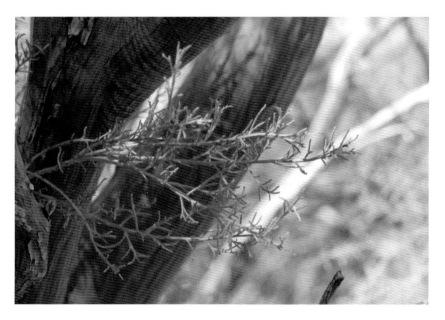

Scientific name – Adenostoma sparsifolium
Common names – Red shank, greasewood, ribbonwood, yerba del pasmo (Spanish)

Identification – Red shank is a large bush, up to 15 feet tall, that grows on dry chapparal slopes in the foothills and low mountains.

The trunk is red-brown. Strips of bark hang off the trunk. The sparse leaves are needle shaped and about half an inch long or less. The flowers are very small, white and grow in sparse bracts (1). Flowers form in the late Spring.

Characteristics – Red shank is a common perennial and may be among the most common species in some areas. It grows at elevations between about 1,000 – 6,000 feet (1). The leaves have very little smell or flavor. The name greasewood indicates the fire hazard from this plant during wild fires. Yerba de pasmo is Spanish for plant of wonder. This indicates that the Spanish may have recognized the medicinal properties of the plant.

Distribution – Red shank is found in the hills and mountains of the central and southern coast of California and into Baja California (1).

Primary uses – A tea can be made from the small branches to treat toothache and to clean wounds and sores. California Indians had a form of sugar that gave them tooth decay and gum disease even before the Europeans arrived. This will be further discussed under Carrizo. The tea has also been used for urinary tract problems and to bathe arthritic limbs (4).

Secondary uses – The tea has been used for sore throat, ulcers, colds, respiratory problems, stomach ache and as a laxative. The seeds of the plant were used as food. A glue was made from the secretions of a scale insect found on the plant. The branches were used as arrow shafts, torches and rabbit sticks (4). Rabbits were frequently hunted with curved rabbit sticks that were thrown like boomerangs.

Active compounds – Adenostoma sparsifolium contains flavonoids and phenolic acids as discussed under A. fasciculatum (5). Some flavonoids may be unique to the leaves of A. sparsifolium. It is not known which flavonoid or phenolic acid in the plant is effective against the bacteria that cause tooth and gum disease.

Recommendation – The tea from this plant has been popular for a long time and can probably be used safely for toothache, sore throat, colds, flus, stomach ache and as a laxative. It can probably be used in conjunction with standard drugs for urinary tract infections. The tea can also be used to clean wounds as a temporary measure. Cleaning wounds is best done with soap and water. Red shank can also be used externally for arthritis pain, provided that standard nonsteroidal anti-inflammatory agents are also used.

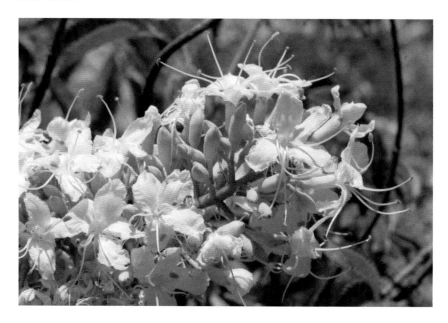

Scientific name – Aesculus californica
Common name – buckeye

Identification – This plant is usually found as a shrub about 10 feet tall, but can grow as a tree up to 36 feet tall. The leaves are about six inches in diameter and divided into a palmate structure of five to seven leaflets. The leaves grow on a large petiole. The flowers grow in an erect panicle of many flowers that looks like a brush and is about six or seven inches long. The flowers are usually white and are about half an inch wide. The fruit, a drupe, looks like a small, brown pear about two inches in diameter and is seen in the fall and early winter. Each drupe contains one large seed (1).

Characteristics – Buckeye can be found along streams or on dry slopes, such as the Tejon Pass area. The nectar and pollen of this plant are reported to be toxic to honey bees (1). Of course, honey bees are not native and come from Europe.

Distribution - The plant is common in Northern and Central California. It grows up to about 5,000 feet in elevation (1).

Primary uses – Buckeye was used as a fish poison. The seeds were ground and put in a dammed stream. The fish would float to the surface and could be collected, cooked and eaten safely. The bark itself or a decoction was used to treat toothaches. Pieces of the seeds were used as suppositories for hemorrhoids (4).

Secondary uses – The seeds of buckeye were used as food during the winter. The seeds were extensively leached before use. In one case, the seeds were roasted in a stone lined pit, ground and placed in a stream to leach for several days. The bark was used as a poultice for wounds and snake bites. The fruit and seeds were used to make poisons (4).

Active compounds – Aesculus seeds are very toxic to mammals and cause muscle paralysis followed by death (6). Extracts of the seeds of an Aesculus species cause brain damage in fish leading to death (7). There are several toxic compounds in Aesculus plants such as sapogenols (8). The seeds contain triterpene oligoglycosides known as escins that have been tested in clinical trials in Europe and Japan, and found to be effective against venous insufficiency, hemorrhoids, and post-operative edema (3, 9). Escins are also anti-inflammatory, as are several sterols found in Aesculus plants. However, escin can also be hepatotoxic and can lower blood glucose (10, 11).

Recommendations – Fish poisons are illegal in the State of California. Given the toxicity of the plant, it is not recommended to use buckeye for toothaches or as a food, unless you have experience with this plant and have eaten it before. The use of a seed as a suppository for hemorrhoids is not safe, since the toxic compounds can be absorbed into the blood from suppositories. Poultices from buckeye are not recommended due to potential toxicity and the fact that they may contain bacteria and fungi. Poisonous snake bites should be treated in a hospital with antivenom. Nonpoisonous snake bites should be washed with soap and water and covered with a clean bandage. It is not recommended to make poisons from this plant.

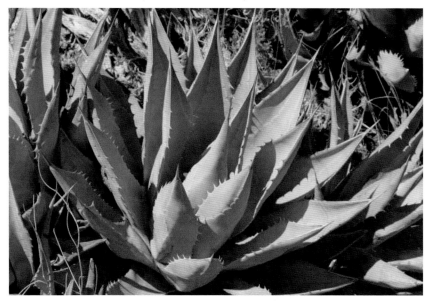

Scientific name – Agave deserti
Common name – Agave, mescal

Identification – The leaves are gray-green, grow in a basal rosette and are about fourteen inches long. The leaves are lanceolate and have teeth along the margins. The flowers grow in a panicle at the top of a stalk that can be up to 12 feet tall. The flowers are light yellow, are tube shaped and have many stamens that exert from the flowers. The flower tubes are about one quarter of an inch long. The fruit are green pods about an inch and a half long (1).

Characteristics – Agave is found in the desert, especially in the desert mountains. It blooms in the Spring (1). This plant has been called mescal for a long time perhaps referring to the use of Agave americana in the production of tequila. Like peyote cactus, also called mescal, it produces a drunken state.

Distribution – The plant is found in the deserts of Southern

California, Arizona and Baja California. It grows in washes and on rocky slopes below 4,500 feet in elevation (1).

Primary uses – Agave was used as a food and a fiber. The stalk was harvested when it was about five feet tall and baked in a stone lined oven in the ground for several days. The flavor is reported to be somewhat sweet and fibrous. The pods were baked in the ovens as well and apparently have a sweet, molasses flavor. The flowers were boiled and eaten. The leaves were also baked and eaten. Fibers were derived from the leaves and are similar to sisal fiber (12). The fibers may have been used for medical purposes such as making casts and securing poultices.

Secondary uses – Soap was sometimes made from the roots by rubbing root scrapings between the palms with water. The sap from agave roots was applied to fresh wounds. The young leaves were chewed as a tonic (4).

Active compounds – Agave contains many compounds including oxalic acid, saponins and triterpenes (13). The sap from Agave americana has been reported to irritate the skin and cause a rash (14). Tequila is distilled from fermented Agave americana, that grows in Mexico.

Recommendations – This is a slowly developing desert plant that should not be harvested in the wild. Please grow it in your garden for personal use. It is safe to eat Agave and use agave fiber. Agave should be baked in a stone oven in the ground as described under Yucca whipplei. It is safe to use soap made from Agave. It is not recommended to put Agave sap on fresh wounds since an irritation may result. The young, uncooked leaves contain saponins that may cause vomiting. Therefore, the young leaves should not be eaten before cooking.

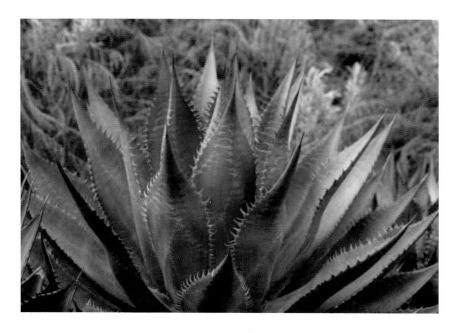

Scientific name – Agave shawii
Common name – Shaw's agave

Identification – The leaves are dark green, grow in a basal rosette and are about sixteen inches long. The leaves are ovate and have teeth along the margins. The flowers grow in a panicle at the top of a stalk that can be 10 feet tall. The flowers are yellow or red, are tube shaped and have many stamens that exert from the flowers. The flower tubes are about three quarters of an inch long. The fruit are green pods about two inches long (1).

Characteristics – The plant blooms in the Spring. It can be purchased from nurseries for growing at home.

Distribution - Shaw's agave is a rare plant that grows on coastal bluffs in San Diego County.

Primary uses – Shaw's agave was used as a food plant as discussed for Agave deserti.

Secondary uses – Fibers were made from the leaves and are

similar to sisal fiber (4). The fibers may have been used for medical purposes such as making casts and securing poultices.

Active compounds – See Agave deserti for a discussion of active compounds.

Recommendations – This is a rare plant that must not be harvested in the wild. It can be grown in your own garden for personal use. It is safe to eat Shaw's agave and use fiber made from this plant. Agave should be baked in a stone oven in the ground as described under Yucca whipplei.

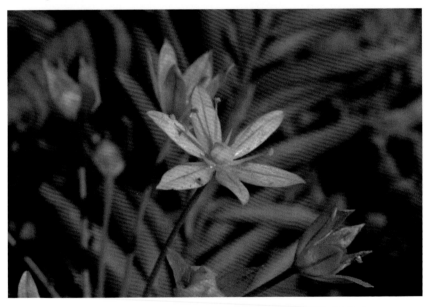

Scientific name – Allium haematochiton
Common name – red skinned onion

Identification – This plant grows from red bulbs about one inch wide. There are from four to six basal leaves that are about six inches long, half an inch wide and are flat. The flowers grow in an umbel on a stem about ten inches tall. There are six petal like structures that are white and make a flower about a third of an inch wide (1).

Characteristics – This is the most common Allium in Southern California. It is found in canyons and grassy areas and is a fire following plant. The leaves smell and taste like onion. It has been very popular as a food and caused the first gold rush in California in 1842. A man harvested some red skinned onions to eat and found gold clinging to the roots. The gold rush area is now called Placerita Canyon.

Distribution – Red skinned onion is found throughout Southern and Baja California. There are several closely related species of Allium, similar to red skinned onion, that occur throughout the West such as Allium amplectens.

Primary uses – The leaves and bulbs of red skinned onion were rubbed on the skin as an insect repellant. The bulbs were rubbed on insect bites to relieve the sting. The crushed bulb was mixed with fat and used to treat snakebite (4).

Secondary uses – The juice from red skinned onion was reduced to a syrup by boiling and used to relieve colds and sore throats. The bulbs were chewed to relieve gas and stimulate the appetite (4).

Active compounds – Allium species contain alliin, ajoene, S-methyl-L-cysteine, flavonoids and other compounds (3). Ajoene inhibits blood clotting. Eating large amounts of Allium plants before surgery can be dangerous due to bleeding problems. Garlic, Allium sativum, is used to control blood pressure and blood cholesterol (3).

Recommendations – It is safe to eat red skinned onions. The Indians harvested them in large amounts and ate them raw or after baking in a stone lined oven in the ground. It is safe to use red skinned onion as an insect repellant and to relieve insect stings. Discontinue use if a rash forms. Do not use this plant against poison snakebites. Instead, go to the emergency room for antivenom treatment. It is safe to use red skinned onion, in moderation, for colds, sore throats, gas and to stimulate the appetite.

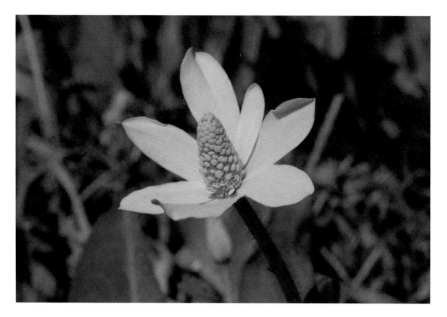

Scientific name – Anemopsis californica
Common names – Yerba mansa (Spanish), swamp root, lizard tail,
'onchoshi (pronounced gonchoeshi, Chumash)

Identification – The plant grows close to the ground and is usually
found growing in colonies. The leaves are oblong, about 3 to 5
inches long and all grow from the base of the plant. The plant
produces a cone of small white flowers. The cone grows on a
stalk about 6 to 10 inches tall. At the base of the cone are 5 to 8
bracts, about an inch long, that look like petals (1).

Characteristics – The plant used to grow near the ocean next to
creeks and sloughs. But this habitat is disappearing quickly. It
blooms from March to September. The late blooms may turn red
or red and white. The plant grows through its rhizomes (roots)
that creep along the ground and establish new plants. The flower
cone is full of tiny, black seeds that taste like pepper. The leaves
also taste peppery and numb the mouth when chewed. The name
yerba mansa means plant of the tame Indians. An Indian who
lived at a Mission was referred to as a Manso (man) or Mansa
(woman). The plant dies back every Summer and regrows from
the roots in the Fall.

24

Distribution – Yerba mansa is found in the western deserts from California to Texas and north to Utah. It grows in saline and alkaline seeps in the desert and foothills (1).

Primary uses – the root of the plant has been used to make a tea for the treatment of venereal diseases, asthma and urinary tract disorders (15, 16, 17). Venereal diseases may have been in California before the Europeans arrived. However, the incidence of these diseases increased dramatically when the Indians lived in the Missions and may have decreased birth rates. The tea is reported to restore strength to the person who drinks it. This plant has been used very widely throughout California (4).

Secondary uses – The root tea was used to wash cuts and sores. It was drunk for the treatment of colds. For arthritis pain, the affected area was soaked in the tea. Toothache was treated by chewing the leaves or seed cone (4, 15).

"In the old days, when a woman became pregnant, she had to think about whether of not she and her baby would be able to survive the winter. Sometimes pregnancies had to be corrected with yerba mansa, California everlasting and tobacco." Cecilia Garcia (Chumash)

Active compounds – Allylveratrole (methyleugenol) is present in the plant and may be responsible for much of the activity of the plant (18). Allylveratrole has been reported to be antispasmodic, which means that is may relax smooth muscles in the bronchi, ureters, gut and other places. The compound also has analgesic activity. Eugenol has been used as a dental pain reliever. A number of flavorful compounds are present such as linalool and thymolmethylether, that may give the plant its peppery taste (19).

Recommendation – This plant has been a very popular remedy in California for a long time and has been reported to be very effective. It is probably safe to use the plant, in moderation, for colds and sores. Cuts should be washed with soap and water and covered with a clean bandage. Yerba mansa can help to numb the mouth during toothaches and is safe to use for this purpose. Simply chew on a leaf. It may be safe to use yerba mansa in addition to standard drugs for the treatment of arthritis and urinary tracts infections. Arthritics should not stop taking nonsteroidal antiinflammatory drugs, but may consider adding yerba mansa to their therapy. Venereal diseases and asthma are serious conditions that should be treated with drugs known to be effective. If you wish to add yerba mansa to your standard therapy for these conditions consult your health care provider. It is not recommended to use any plant preparation to induce abortions. The authors know of no safe preparation to induce abortions. The dose that kills the fetus is usually the dose that kills the mother.

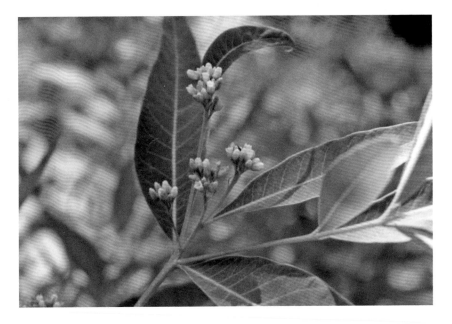

Scientific name – Apocynum cannabinum
Common name – Dogbane, Indian hemp

Identification – This annual plant grows from a single stalk that branches near the top. The leaves are lanceolate, opposite and about three inches long. The flowers are white, urn shaped and about an eighth of an inch long (1).

Characteristics – This plant grows in full shade along streams or wet meadows below 6,000 feet in elevation. It tends to grow in groups and can propogate from the roots.

Distribution – Dogbane is found throughout the Pacific States (2). The habitats this plant grows in are quickly disappearing as water is diverted for city use.

Primary uses – The bark of dogbane was used to make string for many uses, including tying on poultices and casts (4).

Secondary uses – The roots of dogbane were used to treat intestinal and bronchial diseases (4).

Active compounds – Apocynum species contain many flavonoids such as quercetin and hyperoside, an antidepressant (20, 21). Phenylpropanoid favanols, called apocynins, are present and may protect the liver (22). Many glucosides and two pregnane steroids are present (23). Agents active in the heart, called cardenolides are also present (23), and can produce life threatening cardiac arrhythmias or seizures. The cardenolides can be of benefit to people suffering from congestive heart failure, but are toxic to normal people.

Recommendations – It is safe to make cordage from dogbane. It is not recommended to use dogbane preparations internally due to the potential for toxicity. Intestinal and bronchial infections should be treated with drugs known to be effective. Asthma should be treated with drugs known to be effective.

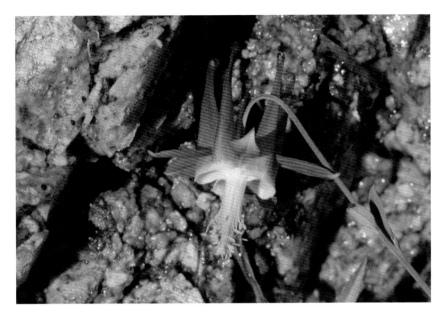

Scientific name – Aquilegia formosa
Common name – crimson columbine

Identification – This plant is usually about two and a half feet tall.
The basal leaves are highly ternately divided. The cauline leaves
are ovate and may be divided into three lobes. The flowers are
nodding and are red and yellow. The flowers are made of five
sepals and five petals. The petals have spurs that project from the
back of the flower (1).

Characteristics – Crimson columbine is found growing beside
mountain streams. It grows below about 9,000 feet in elevation
and is mostly found in pine woodlands (1).

Distribution – This plant is found throughout the Pacific States (2).

Primary uses – A root decoction was used against diarrhea,
stomach ache and indigestion. It was also used against coughs
(4).

Secondary uses – The seeds were used as a diuretic and were
made into a paste with water to treat lice. The entire plant was

used as food after boiling (4).

Active compounds – Aquilegia species contain many alkaloids, cycloartane glycosides and flavonoids (24, 25, 26). Some of the flavonoids such as apigenin and luteolin may be soothing in stomach ache and indigestion.

Recommendations – It is probably safe to use the root of this plant against diarrhea, stomach ache, indigestion and coughs. If diarrhea persists, go to a health care provider for treatment. Please do not collect this beautiful plant in the wild. Grow it in your own garden for personal use. It is probably safe to use the seeds to treat lice and as a short term diuretic. If you need a diuretic for more than a couple of days, consult a health care provider.

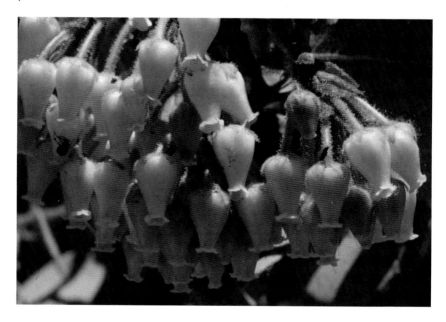

Scientific name – Arctostaphylos glauca
Common name – Manzanita

Identification – This large shrub is usually about six feet tall but can grow to be 24 feet tall. The bark is reddish brown and sometimes peels away from the stem. The leaves are elliptical, about an inch and a half long, have a quarter inch long petiole and may be covered with a fine white powder. The flowers grow in a raceme, are urn shaped, white and about a third of an inch long (1). Flowers form in May and June. The fruit is about half an inch wide, sticky, green and tastes like a golden delicious apple. Inside is a large stone. The fruit forms in July.

Characteristics – Manzanita is the Spanish word for little apple. This species really tastes like an apple if it is eaten before it withers to a brown, dried fruit. This is the most common manzanita species in the mountains of Southern California. It is found in sunny areas of the chaparral and in woodlands below 4,000 feet in elevation.

Distribution – This manzanita grows from the San Francisco bay south into Baja California. However, there are many species of manzanita that grow throughout the West.

Primary uses – The leaves of several manzanita species were made into a decoction and used to treat skin sores, rashes, cuts and bruises. This decoction was also used as a wash to relieve head ache. The decoction was drunk for urinary tract infections (4).

Secondary uses – The berries of some manzanita species were used to stop diarrhea. A decoction made from the berries or leaves was used for bronchial problems (4).

Active compounds – The leaves of Arctostaphylos species contain tannins, flavonoids, triterpenes and other compounds (3). Also present are hydroquinone derivatives such as arbutin that are bacteriostatic in an alkaline environment (3).

Recommendations - Arctostaphylos tea made from uva ursi leaves is widely used in Europe, has been clinically tested in Europe and found to be effective for relief of mild urinary tract infections (3). The tea is usually taken with a small amount of bicarbonate to alkalinize the urine. The Indians would have used lime, made from baking seashells and pounding them into a powder, to alkalinize the urine. This drug cannot be used with cranberry or other preparations that acidify the urine. If the urinary tract infection persists for more than six hours, use an antibiotic agent known to be effective. It is probably safe to use a decoction of manzanita leaves to treat skin problems that are not open. Discontinue use if a rash forms. Open wounds should be treated with soap and water followed by a sterile bandage. It is probably safe to treat head ache with a wash made of the leaves. It is safe to eat the berries, in moderation, to stop diarrhea. Bronchial problems such as asthma or bronchial infections must be treated with drugs known to be effective, not manzanita.

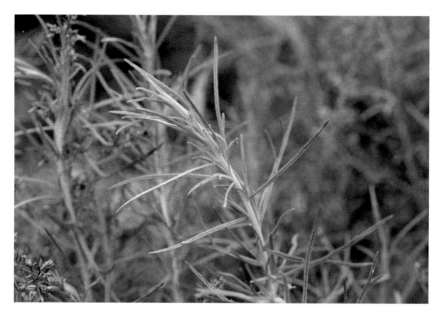

Scientific name – Artemisia californica
Common name – California sagebrush, khapshikh (pronounced kopsheek, Chumash)

Identification – This Artemisia grows as a shrub up to 7 feet high, but usually about 3 feet high, with many branches. The leaves are thread like, light green to silver green and about 2 inches long. The flowers usually form in the fall, are very small and obscured by leaves (1).

Characteristics - California sagebrush grows in chaparral in the foothills and near the coast below 2,500 feet in elevation (1).

The plant has a very strong sagebrush smell and a pungent, moderately bitter, but pleasant taste.

Distribution – This plant grows mostly near the coast from San Francisco to Baja California (1).

Primary uses – California sagebrush was used in girl's puberty rites by the Luiseno and Cahuilla people (4, 27). The skin and clothes were purified and perfumed with the plant. A tea made from the leaves and stems was used by women at the beginning of each menstrual period.

"California sagebrush is used to bring back pleasant memories. Burn it or put it in a sack and smell it to bring back pleasant memories." Cecilia Garcia (Chumash)

Secondary uses – The Costanoans used the leaves for tooth aches and as a poultice for wounds. A decoction of the leaves and stems was used externally for colds, asthma and arthritis. The decoction was drunk for bronchitis. The Cahuilla chewed the leaves and smoked the leaves with Nicotiana attenuata leaves. A necklace of the stems was worn by many California Indians as an insect repellant and to keep evil spirits away (4).

Active compounds - The active compounds in California sagebrush are probably similar to the compounds reported for mugwort. Artecalin, a sesquiterpene lactone of unknown activity, occurs in California sagebrush (28). Artemisia plants are very important medicinal plants throughout the world. They are used against malaria, fungal infections, inflammation, bacterial and viral infections.

Recommendations – It is safe to use California sagebrush to bring back pleasant memories. Familiar, pleasant smells frequently are the best way to bring back pleasant memories. It is safe to use California sagebrush to perfume the skin and clothes. There is no danger, except contact dermatitis, from using California sagebrush preparations externally. If a rash forms, stop using the preparation. A tea made from the stems and leaves can be drunk safely, in moderation, before each period. Bronchitis is frequently a bacterial infection that should be treated with antibiotics. It is not known if California sagebrush has antibiotic activity. It is probably safe to drink a decoction of the leaves for bronchitis, in addition to standard antibiotic drugs. A decoction of the plant can be used safely for colds. Asthma should be treated with standard asthma medications. A California sagebrush decoction can probably be safely added to asthma therapy, in moderation. Arthritis should be treated with anti-inflammatory drugs. A decoction of California sagebrush can probably be added to this in moderation. Nicotiana attenuata should not be used except during rare occasions, since it is addictive. It is not recommended to smoke California sagebrush, since smoking can cause lung damage and emphysema. California sagebrush is a good insect repellant and can be used safely to keep evil spirits away.

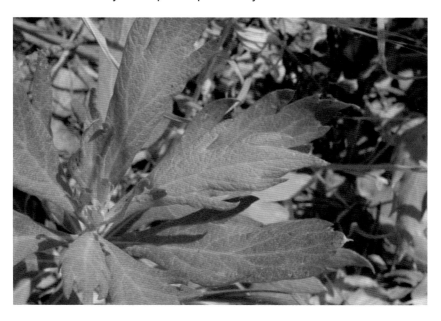

Scientific name – Artemisia douglasiana
Common name – Mugwort, molush (Chumash)

Identification – Mugwort grows to be 7 feet tall, but is usually about 4 feet tall. The stalks are erect with few branches. The leaves are about 4 inches long, oblong and divided into at least 3 lobes. Above, the leaves are dark green. Below, the leaves are white from many hairs. Flowers are very small and are hidden by dense leaves (1).

Characterisics - These plants are found beside or near streams below 6,000 feet in elevation (1). The stems have a mild sage smell and a sweet sage flavor. The leaves smell like sage and have a very bitter flavor. The seeds have a very pungent sage flavor.

Distribution – Mugwort is found from Baja California to Washington and Idaho (1). There are closely related species that grow in Europe and China (3).

Primary uses – Mugwort is a very important medicinal plant with many uses. The leaves of mugwort were chewed to relieve tooth ache pain (4). Tooth and gum diseases are discussed under Carrizo cane. It was also used for menopause, hot flashes, dysmenorrhea and premenstrual syndrome. Mugwort stems and leaves were put under the pillow to promote pleasant dreams. It can even be used by people getting over addictions to help them sleep.

"Mugwort was dream sage, used to neutralize thoughts and let the brain rest. Some people say they can't stop their thoughts and dream. If you can't dream, you can't sleep. It is so vital to health to just go to sleep." Cecilia Garcia (Chumash)

Secondary uses – A tea made from the leaves was used externally to treat poison oak rash and measles (16). However, Chumash people regard mule fat (Baccharis salicifolia) and coyote brush (Baccharis pilularis) as better for poison oak rash (15, 17). The Costanoans used mugwort for urinary tract problems and asthma. A compress was made from the leaves for arthritis. Other California Indians used mugwort for many problems including ear ache, colds, dysentery and to keep evil spirits away (4).

"I rub it before I touch a woman in childbirth. It is the essence of dreams for the mother and child, when I bring life forward. I use it so that their dreams will come true." Cecilia Garcia (Chumash)

Active compounds – This plant contains many active compounds such as cineole, camphor, linalool and other flavors and fragrances (3). Many of these monoterpenoids are pain relievers. Sesquiterpene lactones such as vulgarin and psilostachyin (3) are present and are related to the bitter compounds absinthin and artabsin from wormwood (Artemisia absinthium), the source of absinthe. This plant also contains thujone (3) that induces hallucinations, convulsions and renal damage. Very little thujone is present in teas and other aqueous extracts of Artemisias. Thujone is present in high amounts in alcoholic extracts, as with absinthe. Vincent Van Gogh was an absinthe addict who had vivid hallucinations and convulsions, that lead him to depression and death. Some of his paintings may reflect his hallucinations of objects glowing with an unreal light. Some of the Chumash pictographs may also be representations of objects glowing with an unreal light. Could California Indians have experienced sacred dreams, hallucinations from mugwort? California Indians had alcoholic preparations, wines, that did not contain enough alcohol to extract much thujone. They could have, however, made oil extracts, such as eel oil, that would have contained high concentrations of thujone.

Recommendations – It is best to use a length of mugwort stem as long as the longest finger or a single leaf. This is added to simmering hot water to make a tea for menopause, hot flashes, premenstrual syndrome and dysmenorrhea. This mild tea has a pleasant sage flavor. Sugar should not be added. The seeds have a very strong sage flavor when chewed and have been used to treat dysmenorrhea. Dysmenorrhea should be treated with standard anti-inflammatory drugs, such as naproxen. Mugwort can probably be added to this therapy, in moderation. It may be safe to drink a mild mugwort tea, in moderation, for menopause, hot flashes and premenstrual syndrome. It is also safe to chew on a mugwort leaf for tooth ache pain, from time to time. It is safe to apply a body temperature tea of mugwort leaves to poison oak and measles rashes. However, if the rash becomes worse, this may be a sign of an allergy to mugwort leaves, which means the tea should no longer be used. Arthritis should be treated with anti-inflammatory drugs. Mugwort compresses can be added to standard arthritis therapy. Urinary tract infections and asthma should be treated with drugs known to be effective against these conditions. It is probably safe to add a mild mugwort tea to this therapy. Ear aches and colds can be safely treated by drinking mild mugwort tea, in moderation. Infections of the ear should be treated with standard antibiotic drugs. Dysentery should be treated with drugs known to be effective, not mugwort. Why not use mugwort to keep evil spirits away and promote good dreams? Just put some leaves under the pillow to promote pleasant dreams.

Warning – There are reports of mugwort leaf tea causing abortions (4). It is likely that this involved drinking a large amount of a very strong tea, perhaps over a period of several hours or days. This is very dangerous and would probably kill the mother and the fetus together. Mugwort leaves were used to cauterize wounds. A preparation of dry leaves was placed on the wound and burned (17). This practice left large scars and should not be continued.

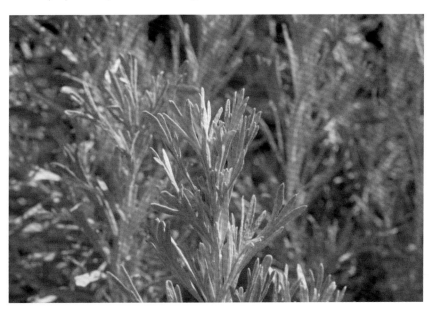

Scientific name – Artemisia tridentata
Common name – Big sagebrush, mountain sagebrush

Identification – This shrub grows from a thick trunk with many branches. The leaves are wedge shaped, usually about one half of an inch long and have three lobes. They are gray green and densely hairy. As with other Artemisias, the flowers are very small and hidden by leaves (1).

Characteristics - This plant is common and grows in dry areas up to 9,000 feet in elevation. The leaves have a strong smell of sagebrush.

Distribution – This plant grows throughout the Western US and Northern Mexico (1).

Primary uses – Big sagebrush was used in the sweat lodge to purify the air. A preparation of powdered leaves was used for chafing. The Paiute and Kawaiisu used the leaves or an infusion of the leaves to cure colds and stomach aches (4, 29, 30).

Secondary uses – A tea made from the leaves was used as a disinfectant wash. The leaves were used as a poultice by many California Indians (4).

Active compounds – Big sagebrush contains several coumarins including 7-methylesculin, esculin, umbelliferone and others (31). Some coumarins are anticoagulants or relax smooth muscle. Also present are flavonoids such as luteolin, axillarin and eupafolin (31). Many monoterpenes have been found in big sagebrush (32). Monoterpenes give the plant most of its smell and flavor. Artevasin, a sesquiterpene lactone, has been identified in the plant (33). Sesquiterpene lactones can have antimicrobial, antitumor and other activities.

Recommendations – It is safe to use this plant, in moderation, for aroma therapy, to purify the air, against chafing, for colds and stomach aches. If a rash forms when using the plant against chafing, stop using the preparation since this may indicate an allergy. It is best to use a preparation of known disinfectant activity, rather than big sagebrush, since its disinfectant activity has not been tested. In general poultices can be used as temporary bandages until a more sterile bandage can be applied. Poultices can place bacteria and fungi from the plant into an open wound. If a temporary poultice is applied, make sure to use an antibiotic compound on the wound as soon as possible and replace the poultice with a sterile bandage. Always wash open wounds with soap and water.

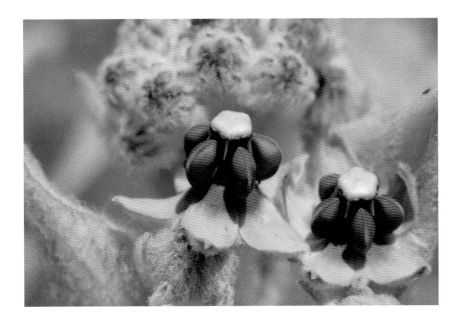

Scientific name – Asclepias californica
Common names – California milkweed, round hooded milkweed

Identification – The stems and leaves of this small shrub are densely hairy. The plant grows to about 2 feet tall. The leaves are ovate with a short petiole. The flowers have white or pink petals that are reflexed. The flower hoods are purple with white spots (1).

Characteristics and Distribution – This plant is found in dry, sunny areas up to 6,000 feet in elevation. It is found from the Sierra Nevada mountains to Baja California (2). Occasionally, monarch larvae can be found eating this milkweed.

Primary use – The Kawaiisu used this milkweed to treat spider bites. The leaves were dried, pulverized and applied as a poultice (4).

Secondary use – The sap of this milkweed was dried and chewed as gum, which may have helped clean the teeth and gums (4, 30). Tooth and gum decay were a serious concern of many California

Indians as discussed under Carrizo cane.

Active compounds – Most or all milkweed species contain ouabain, a toxic cardiac glycoside and similar cardenolides (34). Overdosing with ouabain can lead to cardiac arrhythmias and death. The flowers and leaves of various Asclepias species contain flavonoids, steroidal glycosides, megastigmane glucosides, and several phenolic compounds (35, 36, 37, 38). Monarch butterflies are stimulated to lay their eggs by the presence of the proper flavonol glycoside in the Asclepias species (39).

Recommendation – It is safe to use this plant as a temporary poultice for the bites of nonpoisonous spiders after washing the bite with soap and water. Steroidal glycosides in the plant may enhance the healing of these bites. The poultice may contain bacteria and fungi and should be replaced with a clean bandage as soon as possible. However, be aware that the bite of the brown recluse spider is best treated in a hospital. Serious damage and even death can result from improperly treated brown recluse spider bites. Black widow spider bites are best treated by a health care provider, although they are rarely life threatening. Due to the probable presence of ouabain and other cardiac glycosides in this plant, chewing a gum made from the sap is not recommended. Ouabain is toxic and can cause death from cardiac arrhythmias. It is safer to use a tooth brush for dental hygiene.

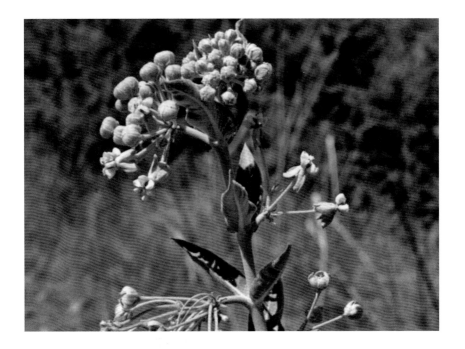

Scientific name – Asclepias erosa
Common name – Desert milkweed

Identification – This plant grows on tall stems, up to 5 feet tall, that usually are not hairy. The leaves grow opposite each other on the stem and have no petioles. They are usually elliptical. The flowers have reflexed, white petals, with cream colored or yellow hoods. The hoods usually have horns (1).

Characteristics – This plant is a great favorite of the tarantula hawk (Pepsis thisbe). The female wasps are an inch and a half long and greedily seek out this plant and Asclepias subulata for nectar. The adult wasps drink nectar. The wasp larvae eat paralyzed tarantulas. Beware the sting of the tarantula hawk. It is rated as one of the most painful stings from an American wasp.

Distribution - This milkweed is found in desert canyons up to 6,000 feet in elevation (1, 2). It is found from the southern San Joaquin Valley of California to Arizona and Baja California.

Primary use – The sap of this milkweed was heated by the fire and dried into a gum (4). Chewing this gum may have promoted dental hygiene. California Indians suffered from tooth and gum decay as discussed under Carrizo cane.

Secondary use - The Tubatulabal used the sap of this milkweed to treat sores and rashes caused by poison oak (4).

Active compounds – These are discussed under Asclepias californica.

Recommendation – It is probably safe to use the sap of this plant externally to treat sores and rashes. Steroidal compounds in the plant may promote healing of rashes and sores. Discontinue use if the rash gets worse or a new rash forms. It is not recommended to chew gum made from the sap of this milkweed, since this plant probably contains ouabain and other cardiac glycosides. These poisonous compounds can cause cardiac arrhythmias that can be fatal. A tooth brush is a safer way to clean the teeth.

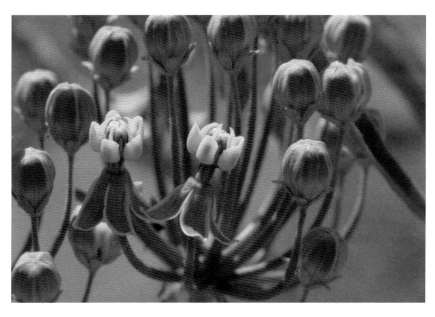

Scientific name – Asclepias fascicularis
Common names – Narrow leaf milkweed, tok (pronounced toke,

Chumash)

Identification – The stalks of this annual plant have few branches and can grow to be 4 feet high. The leaves are narrowly lanceolate, about 3 inches long and may grow in clusters. The flowers are usually white with a pink tinge and grow in umbels (1). When cut, the stem exudes milky, white sap. The plant has little smell, except for the flowers that can have a mild, sweet smell like honey.

Characteristics – Narrow leaf milkweed is highly favored by monarch butterfly larvae, milkweed aphids and milkweed bugs. Monarch caterpillars sometimes eat the plant down to the bare stalk. This plant should be protected in order to protect the California populations of monarch butterflies. Unfortunately, monarch butterfly populations have been dwindling for many years due to destruction of milkweed habitats.

Distribution - The plant is found throughout the Pacific States in dry, sunny areas up to 6,000 feet in elevation (2).

Primary uses – This plant was a good source of fibers for cordage (4, 30). Milkweed cordage was used to bind together splints (see Tule) and to hold poultices in place. Cordage produced from milkweed is not as high quality as cordage made from Apocynum.

Secondary uses – The pods, flowers, leaves, shoots and roots were used as food and are reported to taste like mild asparagus (4). The plant was boiled three times in three changes of water before eating. The leaves were used as a poultice for snake bites. The fresh flowers were used as a poison. The Yokuts mixed the sap of this plant with oil from Marah fabaceus seeds and added this binder to pigments to make paints for pictographs. The sap of this milkweed was used by the Cahuilla as an adhesive (27). The sap was dried and chewed as gum by many California Indians, especially when combined with deer or salmon fat (4). Chewing unsweetened gum may have aided dental hygiene. Salmon used to run in California rivers as far south as Point Conception. Legends state that the salmon will return every year if God is pleased with the people. Salmon runs are virtually extinct in California now.

Active compounds – Refer to Asclepias californica.

Recommendation – It is safe to use milkweed for cordage. The bark is stripped from the plant and rolled between the palms or on the thigh to produce fibers. Two or three fibers are wound into strings. It is potentially dangerous to eat milkweed or chew milkweed gum. However, it is possible that carefully boiling it three times, and throwing out the water after each boiling, may remove most of the poisonous ouabain. For dental hygiene, it is safer to use a tooth brush than to chew milkweed gum. It is not safe to make a poultice for rattlesnake bite, which should be treated in a hospital with antivenom. For the bites of nonpoisonous snakes, wash the area with soap and water and apply a temporary poultice if desired. The poultice may contain bacteria and fungi and should be replaced with a clean bandage as soon as possible. Look at the bite several times each day to make sure there is no infection. Minor infections should be treated by applying an antibiotic ointment or see a health care provider. It is safe to use the sap as an adhesive. It is not recommended to use the flowers as a poison.

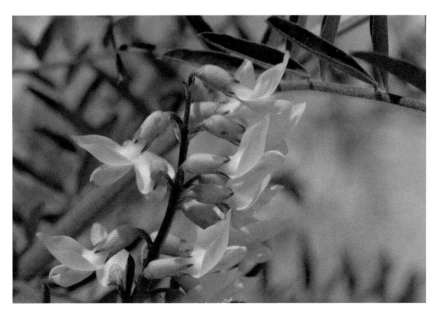

Scientific name – Astragalus pomonensis
Common name – Milk vetch

Identification – This is a low lying plant that is usually about eight inches tall. The branches are spreading. The leaves are pinnately divided into 25-41 elliptical leaflets about half an inch long. The flowers grow in a dense raceme, are white and resemble pea flowers. The pods are bladdery and about an inch and a half long (1).

Characteristics – Milk vetch grows in grassy areas below about 2,000 feet in elevation. There are many Astragalus species in Southern California. This one is probably the most common. This genus contains loco weed, which annually kills many cows. However, many Astragalus species are referred to as milk vetch and are safe for cows to eat.

Distribution – This plant is localized to Southern California from San Luis Obispbo to San Bernardino (2). However, there are many similar milk vetch species that occur throughout the west.

Primary uses – Some Astragalus species were used as food, especially the pods that were eaten as a food and spice (4).

Secondary uses – Astragalus purshii and Astragalus pachypus were used by the Kawaiisu to relieve menstrual pain (4). A decoction of the roots was drunk and was reported to cause an intoxication similar to Datura wrightii (4). Meat, fat and salt were not eaten for a month after drinking the decoction.

Active compounds – Astragalus species contain many active compounds including cycloartane type triterpene glycosides that are in part responsible for the plants' immunostimulatory activity (40). However, some Astragalus species, usually the ones called locoweed, contain swainsonine and perhaps other toxic agents (41). Poisoning from Astragalus involves chronic ingestion over the period of several days or weeks and is most common in horses, cows and sheep. The animals may develop tremors, become paralyzed and die.

Recommendations – It is not recommended to eat any Astragalus

44

plant or drink decoctions of Astragalus. This is because it is difficult to know which species contain toxic agents, and which do not. There are many different species of Astragalus in California, many of which are difficult to identify. Any species that produces an intoxication of the brain should be avoided, since this may indicate the presence of swainsonine. The Chinese have used Astragalus for many years as an immunostimulant. Perhaps it is most advisable to buy a preparation of Astragalus that is known to be safe.

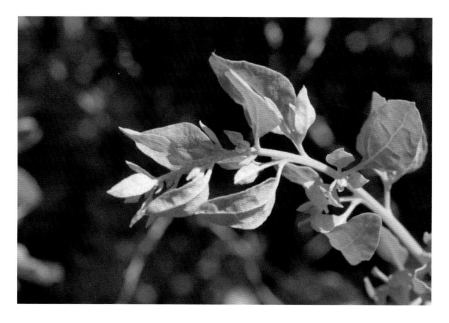

Scientific name – Atriplex lentiformis
Common name – Big saltbush, quail bush

Identification – This shrub is usually about four feet tall. The highly variable leaves are about three quarters of an inch long and have gray scales. They can be ovate, deltate or hastate (1) and have a salty flavor. The flowers are so small, they are usually not seen. The brown seeds are prominent in long clumps at the ends of the branches. The seeds form in April and May. The seeds taste like popcorn, complete with a light salty flavor, but no butter.

Characteristics – Big saltbush is found in coastal marshes

and other marshes below 4,500 feet in elevation. Coastal environments are rapidly being developed into housing and shopping areas at the expense of big saltbush. The seeds of big saltbush and desert Atriplex species were very important as food (4). The cicadas that are found on desert Atriplex bushes were eaten as well.

Distribution – This plant is found from central California to Utah and Mexico (1). Other Atriplex species are found throughout the west.

Primary uses – Colds were treated by chewing the leaves or smoking the dried leaves of an Atriplex species. Alternatively, the steam from boiling leaves and stems was inhaled to help against colds and nasal congestion (4).

Secondary uses – Atriplex roots were used to treat wounds, ant bites and skin infections. Atriplex was used by the Kumeyaay against pain (4).

Active compounds – Atriplex species contain triterpenes, sterols, phytoecdysteroids and other compounds (42). Phytoecdysteroids are toxic to insects and protect the seeds of Atriplex and other plants from insect damage. Phytoecdysteroids prevent moulting in insects but appear to not be especially toxic to man.

Recommendations – It is safe to eat the seeds of big saltbush. It is probably safe to eat cicadas also. It is probably safe to treat colds by chewing the leaves or inhaling the steam from boiling big saltbush. It is not recommended to smoke the leaves since smoking anything damages the lungs. It is probably safe to use the leaves against ant bites and pain, in moderation. It is not recommended to use the leaves on wounds or infections. These are best treated with soap, water, antibiotics and sterile bandages. Skin infections may be best treated by a health care provider.

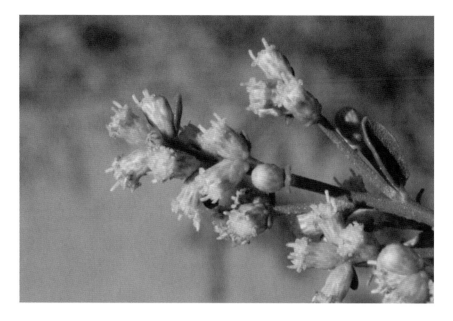

Scientific name – Baccharis pilularis
Common name – Coyote Brush

Identification – This large shrub grows to about eight feet tall. The leaves have very short petioles, are about half an inch long, are oval and have many teeth along the margins. The small flowers grow in bell shaped heads, about a quarter of an inch long, with prominent white bristles (1).

Characteristics – This common plant is found near the coast and inland in oak woodlands to about 2,000 feet in elevation. It prefers moist areas and can be common.

Distribution – The plant is found from Oregon to Northern Mexico (1)

Primary uses – Coyote brush was used as a leaf decoction to treat poison oak rash. The Chumash use this plant as the primary poison oak treatment (15). The leaves were also used as poultices for wounds and skin problems.

Secondary uses – Coyote brush was a general remedy for many illnesses, especially when the preferred plant was not available.

Active compounds – Baccharis species contain flavones, diterpenes, monoterpenes and other compounds (43, 44, 45). Some of the diterpenes, such as gaudichaudol and articulin, are cytotoxic against cancer cells (46). Some Brazilian and Argentinian Baccharis species contain highly toxic macrocyclic trichothecenes that poison cattle (47). Baccharis species contain anti-inflammatory, antibiotic, antifungal and antiviral compounds (43, 45, 48).

Recommendations – It is safe to use coyote brush to treat poison oak rash. Discontinue use if the rash does not clear up within a week. Do not use this plant as a poultice for wounds since the leaves may introduce bacteria and fungi into the wound. Wounds should be treated with soap, water and a clean bandage. Coyote brush should be used with caution internally since it may contain toxic compounds.

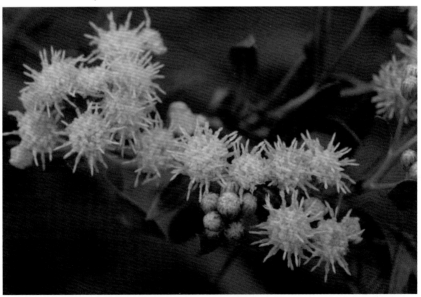

Scientific name – Baccharis salicifolia
Common name – Mule fat

Identification – This plant grows from several long stems and resembles willow. It grows to about ten feet tall. The leaves are lanceolate and about three inches long. The flowers grow in a panicle of cone shaped heads containing very small flowers and white bristles. The heads are about a third of an inch long (1).

Characteristics – This common plant grows in moist canyons and along streams. It grows below 4,000 feet in elevation. In some areas there may be a summer form and a winter form of the plant, which do not look exactly alike (1). Mule fat sticks were the preferred fire drills for many Indians (4).

Distribution – Mule fat is found from Northern California to Texas and South America (1).

Primary uses – The leaves were made into an infusion to wash the hair, promote hair growth and prevent baldness (4, 27).

Secondary uses – A tea made from the leaves was used as a feminine hygiene agent and an eye wash (4, 27).

Active compounds – See Baccharis pilularis for a full discussion. Apparently, mule fat does not contain toxic trichothecenes. The name mule fat comes from the fact that gold miners fed the plant to their mules to keep them fat.

Recommendations – It is safe to use mule fat as a hair wash and treatment, especially if it prevents baldness. It is probably safe to use a leaf tea for feminine hygiene, in moderation, to help control external yeast and bacteria. Discontinue use if a rash forms. It is not recommended to use this plant as an eye wash. Only sterile solutions should be put onto the eye.

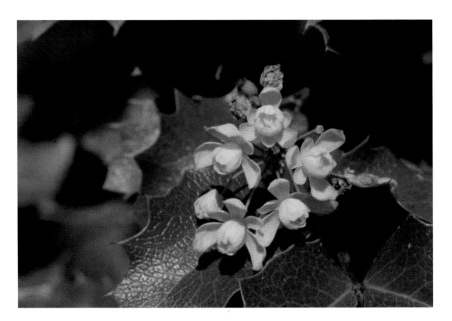

Scientific name – Berberis aquifolium
Common name – Oregon grape

Identification – This plant can grow as a low, spreading plant or a
bush up to 6 feet tall. The leaves can be dark green or red, and
grow in a pinnate formation of 5-9 leaflets. The leaflets are round
or elliptical and are about two inches long or more. The edges of
the leaflets have teeth tipped with spines. The yellow flowers grow
in a raceme. Each flower is about a quarter of an inch in diameter.
The fruit is usually purple and nearly half an inch in diameter (1).
The fruit does have a flavor similar to grapes, although not nearly
as sweet.

Characteristics – Oregon grape is found throughout California,
although it is less common south of Santa Barbara. It is found in
canyons, forests and chaparral below about 6,000 feet in elevation
(1).

Distribution – This plant is widely distributed from Canada to the
Great Plains to Mexico (1).

Primary uses – The Kawaiisu used a decoction of the roots to treat gonorrhea (4). Venereal diseases may have occurred in California before the Spanish arrived, but greatly increased when the Indians were forced to live at the Missions.

Secondary uses – The inner bark or roots were used to make a tea to stimulate the appetite (4). The berries were fermented to make a wine.

'Wine was used for relaxation during the challenge of story telling. We had an oral history. But a lot of trades were silent, especially hunters. People didn't waste their words. When people gathered, the words had to come out. It was time to share knowledge." Cecilia Garcia (Chumash)

Active compounds – Berberine is discussed under Berberis nevinii and is an antimicrobial agent that has not been tested against gonorrhea. Berberine is also an anti-inflammatory since it can decrease cyclooxygenase 2 activity making it potentially useful in arthritis (49). Berberis fruit has antihistamine activity (50), which may relieve indigestion.

Recommendations – Venereal diseases are best prevented. A health care provider should treat venereal diseases. Gonorrhea is usually cured quickly. However, discuss with your health care provider adding Berberis to your therapy. Most people do not need to stimulate their appetite. However, indigestion may be safely and pleasantly treated with Berberis fruit, in moderation. It is safe to drink one glass of wine a day, not more. Excessive drinking leads to heart disease, gut problems and liver disease. Sharing knowledge is essential to the future of our society.

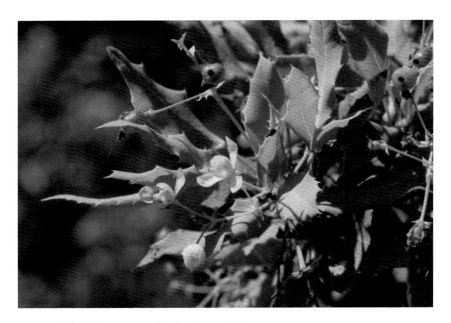

Scientific name – Berberis nevinii
Common name – Nevin's barberry

Identification – This bush can grow to be 12 feet tall, but is usually about 4 feet tall.   The leaves grow in a pinnate formation of 3-5 leaflets. The leaflets are about an inch and a half long. The gray-green leaflets are narrow, elliptical and have spine tipped teeth. The small, yellow flowers grow in a raceme. The spherical fruit is about a quarter of an inch in diameter and is red (1).

Characteristics – This is an endangered species. It used to be found in washes and chaparral areas below 2,000 feet in elevation (1). Habitat destruction and introduced species may contribute to the loss of this plant in the wild.

Distribution – This rare plant is only found in Southern California, not far from the coast (1).

Primary uses – A Berberis root decoction was used to treat tuberculosis (4). The species used may have been B. pinnata rather than B. nevinii.

Secondary uses – The roots of this and most Berberis species were used to make a yellow dye for basket work. The fruit of most Berberis species were eaten raw or cooked by most Indians (4).

Active compounds – Berberine is an isoquinoline alkaloid found in the roots and bark of Berberis species. Berberine has a wide range of antimicrobial activity. Berberis plants also contain 5'-methoxyhydnocarpin that greatly increases the antimicrobial activity of berberine (51). Berberine is also effective against malaria plasmodia (52).

Recommendations – Tuberculosis may have occurred in California before Europeans arrived. The disease greatly increased in the Missions. Tuberculosis is a disease that appears to be increasing in some inner city populations. The disease can be difficult to cure. Tuberculosis should be treated by a health care provider. Ask your health care provider about adding Berberis to your therapy. Berberis nevinii is endangered and should not be collected in the wild. However, you can grow it in your garden after purchasing the plant from a nursery. New drugs for tuberculosis and malaria are a constant need. Perhaps Berberis plants will one day give us new drugs for these diseases.

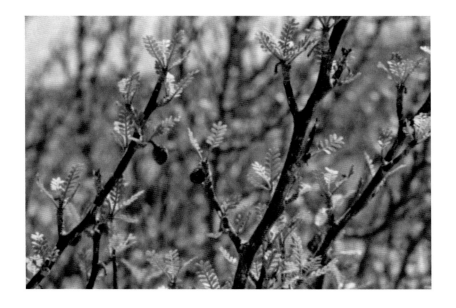

Scientific name – Bursera microphylla
Common name – Elephant tree, torote (Spanish)

Identification – This desert tree grows to about twelve feet tall
with spreading branches that are usually reddish brown. The
leaves are pinnately divided into 7-33 leaflets that are about a
quarter of an inch long. The flowers are about a quarter of an inch
across and have about five white petals. The fruit is dark brown,
has three valves, yellow seeds and is about a third of an inch in
diameter (1).

Characteristics – This is a rare, slow growing desert plant that
must not be harvested in the wild. It grows on rocky slopes below
2,000 feet in elevation in the Sonora Desert of San Diego County
(1). The fruit tastes like a sweet orange.

Distribution – Elephant tree is rare in California and more common
in Arizona and Mexico, in the Sonoran Desert (1). In fact, elephant
tree was unknown in California until 1937 (4). However, there are
several species of Bursera that occur in Arizona and Mexico that
were extensively used as medicines (53).

Primary uses – The sap of elephant tree was rubbed on skin diseases and sores (4).

Secondary uses – The sap (copal) was considered to be supernaturally powerful and could give someone power over another person, such as when gambling (4). Mexican people historically used Bursera for many conditions (53).

Active compounds – Bursera plants contain triterpenoid lactones, flavonoids and other compounds (54, 55). Bursera plants have anti-inflammatory and antihemorrhagic activities (56). However, a number of cytotoxic compounds are present in Bursera plants such as sapelins and many lignans including deoxypodophyllotoxin, burseran and others (57, 58). These cytotoxic agents may be responsible for the spermicidal activity of Bursera extracts (59). Podophyllotoxin, chemically very similar to deoxypodophyllotoxin, causes fetal malformations.

Recommendations – This slow growing, rare desert tree is best left alone. The presence of potentially toxic compounds in the plant makes internal use not advisable.

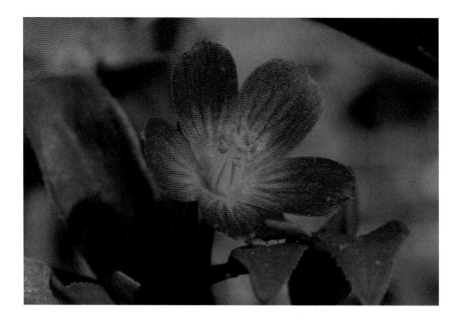

Scientific name – Calandrinia ciliata
Common name – red maids, khutash (Chumash)

Identification – This small, spreading plant grows close to the ground. The leaves are fleshy, oblanceolate and about two inches long. The flowers have five petals and are about a third of an inch wide. The petals are red with white lines (1).

Characteristics – This is a fire following plant that is much more abundant in the year after a fire. It tends to grow in grassy areas below about 6,000 feet in elevation (1). This plant is being largely displaced by non-native grasses introduced by cattle ranchers. It blooms mostly in March and April.

Distribution – Red maids are found throughout the Pacific states (2).

Primary uses – The seeds, flowers, leaves and stems of red maids were eaten and were an important Spring food (4). The leaves have a grassy flavor. The seeds can be toasted with hot rocks in a basket (60). The basket must be moved constantly to avoid scorching the basket. The toasted seeds have a pleasant, toasted nut flavor reminiscent of toasted black sesame seeds. Many Indians grew red maids in their fields and increased the crop by burning their fields every year (15).

Secondary uses – The Chumash used the seeds as offerings to the sun (15). The offerings were usually made at hot springs, which were shrines. Khutash also means earth goddess.

Active compounds – There have been no investigations reported of the active compounds of red maids.

Recommendations – It is safe to eat and enjoy red maids plants and seeds, in moderation. Please do not gather the plants in the wild. You can buy the seeds from seed suppliers and grow them at home. It is safe to make offerings to God. However, perhaps all of the sacred hot springs have been desecrated.

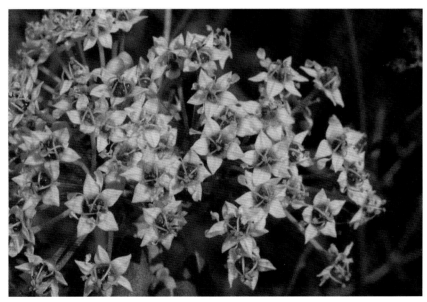

Scientific name – Ceanothus crassifolius
Common name – Hoaryleaf ceanothus

Identification – This bush grows to be as much as 11 feet tall. The twigs are covered with hairs, that are usually white. The one inch long leaves grow opposite each other on the stem, are elliptical and dark green. The evergreen leaves are one ribbed and usually have small teeth on the margins. The upper surface has no hair, whereas the lower surface is covered with hair. The small, white flowers grow in racemes (1).

Characteristics – This common bush is found in many chaparall and canyon areas. It is most common in shaded areas below 3,000 feet in elevation (1).

Distribution – Hoary leaf ceanothus grows from Santa Barbara county to northern Baja California (1).

Primary uses – Hoaryleaf ceanothus was used to stop bleeding. The bark itself or a tea made by boiling the bark was put on open wounds to stop bleeding (4).

Secondary uses – The flowers and young seed pods were used to make a lather that was used as a soap or shampoo (4). This was done by rubbing the flowers between the palms with water. The wood of this and other Ceanothus species was used to make digging sticks (61). The sticks were weighted with circular pieces of soapstone with holes in the middle, and resembled donuts. These digging sticks were used for digging up roots and for other purposes. The roots of this and other Ceanothus species were used to make a red dye for basketry (4).

Active compounds - Ceanothus plants contain many alkaloids and flavonoids (62). Unusual cylopeptide alkaloids, called phenyl cyclopeptines, are present in the bark including integerressin, integerrenin, integerrin and americine (63, 64, 65). The flowers and leaves contain flavonol anthocyanins including derivatives of delphinidin, kaempferol and quercitin (34). Some Ceanothus species (34) contain nonacosane, hexacosanol, velutin, betulinic acid and methylsalicylate (an analgesic). Recently triterpenes were identified in a species of Ceanothus that demonstrate antimicrobial activity against oral pathogens (66). These triterpenes include maesopsin and the antimicrobial compounds ceanothic acid and ceanothetric acid.

Recommendations – The best way to stop bleeding is direct pressure with the hands to the bleeding area. The pressure should be continued until the bleeding stops, even if this requires 10 or 20 minutes. If protective gloves are available, put on the gloves before applying pressure. Looking around for some Ceanothus to make an extract and stop the bleeding is potentially dangerous since the time required may be very bad for the person bleeding. It is safe and advisable to use this plant as soap and shampoo. Thorough washing can help against skin and hair problems as well as insect infestations.

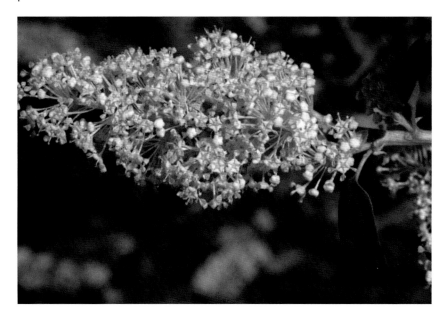

Scientific name – Ceanothus integerrimus
Common name – Deer brush

Identification – This widely distributed bush grows to be about 12 feet tall. The twigs are usually pale green. The deciduous leaves grow alternately on the stem, are about two inches long and are usually lanceolate. The upper surface is light green. The lower surface is lighter green. The small, pale blue or white flowers grow in large racemes (1).

Characteristics – This plant is found in dry, sunny areas where it can be the dominant plant. It is found between 1,000 and 6,000 feet in elevation (1). Flowers appear in May and June.

Distribution – Deer brush is found in the Pacific states (1).

Primary uses – Deer brush was used to treat colds, fevers and stomach aches (4). Kidney, liver and blood diseases were also treated with this plant (4). California Indians thought that impurities in the blood were sometimes the cause of poor health. Purifying the blood involved exercise and purgatives. Probably deer brush was used as a purgative to purify the blood.

Secondary uses – A decoction was made of deer brush to treat facial blemishes (4). The plant was used to make both tonics and sedatives (4). The flowers were used to make soap and shampoo simply by rubbing the flowers between the palms with water (4). Rattles were made from the cocoons of silkworm moths, called ceanothus moths (Hyalophora euryalus, Saturniidae) that live on this and other Ceanothus species as well as Cercocarpis betuloides, Salix species, Arctostaphylos species and Ribes species.

Active compounds – Refer to C. crassifolius.

Recommendations – It is probably safe to use deer brush to treat colds, flus and stomach aches. High fevers should be treated with aspirin or other drugs known to help against fever. Be very careful to use only the dose recommended of the drug, and not more. It is probably safe to use a strong tea made from the bark of deer brush as a laxative. Kidney and liver diseases are serious conditions that should be treated by a health care provider. Discuss with your health care provider the possibility of adding deer brush to your therapy for these conditions. It is safe to use this plant as a soap and shampoo. It is probably safe to make a weak tea of the bark to use, in moderation, as a tonic and sedative. Tonics are drugs that restore normal tissue tone.

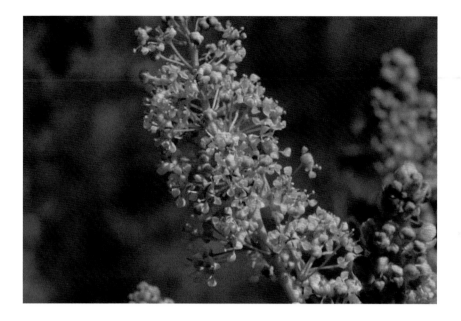

Scientific name – Ceanothus leucodermis
Common name – Chaparral whitethorn

Identification – This thorny bush grows to be about 12 feet tall.
The twigs are covered with gray powder. The evergreen leaves
are about 1 inch long, elliptical and have 3 ribs. The small flowers
grow in racemes and are white or pale blue (1).

Characteristics – This ceanothus grows in dry, sandy or rocky
areas below about 5,000 feet in elevation (1).

Distribution – Chaparral whitethorn occurs from the San Francisco
Bay west to the Sierra Nevada foothills and south to northern Baja
California (1).

Primary uses – A tea was made from the bark and roots and used
as a general tonic, to restore tissue tone (4).

Secondary uses – The berry was boiled to make a tea that was
applied to skin irritations, sores and to stop itches (4). The
blossoms and leaves were crushed and applied to skin irritations

(4). The berries were used to make lather by rubbing them between the palms with water. This lather was used as shampoo and soap. The flowers were also used to make a shampoo (4).

Active compounds – These are discussed under C. crassifolius.

Recommendations – It is probably safe to make a weak tea of the bark to use, in moderation, as a tonic. It is safe to use the berries and flowers to make lather for washing. Daily washing was very important to many California Indians, including the Chumash who bathed everyday before the sun rose. Of course, this was not allowed at the Missions. This may be why skin diseases and insect infestations became more prominent in the Missions.

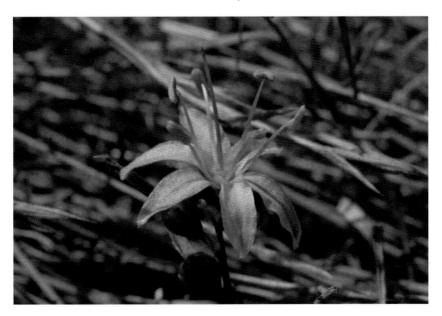

Scientific name – Chlorogalum parviflorum
Common names – small soap plant

Identification – This plant grows from a bulb that is about two inches in diameter and covered with brown membranes. The leaves are about 3/8 of an inch wide, up to six inches long and have very wavy margins. The flowers form only after sufficient rain and are born by a stem that is about two feet high. There are six white or pinkish petals that are reflexed and are about half an inch long. The flowers are open during daylight, but only for one day (1). They form in May and June.

Characteristics – This plant grows in dry, open areas such as ridges in the foothills and coastal scrub below 2,500 feet in elevation (1). This plant is common in the hills of San Diego County, and blooms in May.

Distribution – This plant is only found in the San Diego County, Orange County and northern Baja California coastal areas (1).

Primary uses – The Kumeyaay people used the bulb of small soap plant for soap and shampoo (67). Shampoos were very important for controlling flea and lice infestations.

Secondary uses – The bulb was eaten after extensive boiling in several changes of water (30, 67). The flavor is not reported to be particularly good.

Active compounds – This plant contains saponins that are good detergents (68).

Recommendations – It is safe and recommended to use this plant as a soap and shampoo. This is a slowly proliferating plant that tends to regrow every year from its bulb. Small soap plant should be grown at home for personal use. This plant can be cooked in a stone lined oven, as described under Yucca whipplei, prior to eating. Inadequate cooking can lead to diarrhea.

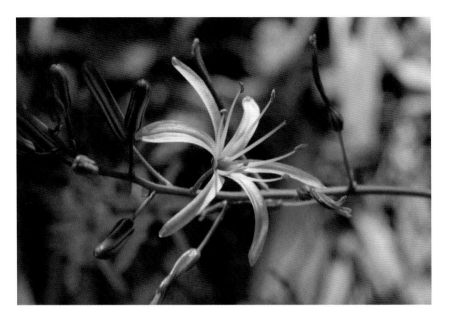

Scientific name – Chlorogalum pomeridianum
Common names – soap plant, amole (Spanish), pash (Chumash)

Identification – This plant grows from a bulb that is about four inches in diameter and covered with brown fibers. The leaves can be up to two and a half feet long and are about half an inch wide. The margins are somewhat wavy. The flowers grow in wide panicles on stems that are up to eight feet tall (1). The flowers are beautiful and white with six slender petals that are about an inch long. They open about 7:00 PM and close before the next morning by wrapping the petals together in a screw like formation. Flowers form from March to July.

Characteristics – Soap plant is usually found in canyons and sheltered valley grasslands below 4,500 feet in elevation (1). It is a fire following plant and grows from seeds after a fire.

Distribution – The plant is found throughout California and southwest Oregon (1).

Primary uses – The bulb of soap plant was used to make shampoo and soap. The soap was used to wash sores, wounds, rashes and feverish people (4). The Chumash and other people bathed and washed with a plant derived soap every day before the sun rose. When they went to the Missions, bathing was not allowed. Skin and scalp problems became common in the Missions (15) due to this lack of bathing.

Secondary uses – The bulbs of soap plant were used as a fish poison (4). The crushed bulbs were placed in a dammed stream. The fish floated to the surface and were cooked prior to eating. The bulbs were eaten by many California Indians after extensive baking in a stone lined oven in the ground (4, 69). The young shoots were also eaten after roasting. The bulbs were used to make a decoction that was a laxative and diuretic (4). The fibers from the bulb were used to make brushes that were used for many purposes, including brushing the hair (4). The bulbs were roasted over a fire in a steatite bowl to produce a glue (4) that may have been mixed with asphaltum and pine sap in order to make a hot glue. This glue was used for many purposes, such as gluing casts together and gluing the boards of plank canoes together. Casts are discussed under tule (Scirpus acutus).

Active compounds – Chlorogalum plants contain saponins that are good detergents and are toxic to fish (68).

Recommendations – It is safe and recommended to use soap plant as a soap and shampoo. This plant can be purchased at many nurseries and can be easily grown at home. Washing wounds, sores and rashes with soap plant and water is recommended. Wounds should be covered with a clean bandage after washing. Washing feverish people is also recommended as this can help bring down a fever. Use of fish poison is illegal in the state of California. Eating the soap plant bulb requires extensive cooking, such as in a stone lined oven as described under Yucca whipplei. Improper cooking may lead to diarrhea. It is not recommended to use this plant orally, except in very small amounts, as a laxative or diuretic since saponins can be toxic in high doses. It is safer to use this plant as an enema for its laxative effect and avoid oral use. It is safe and recommended to use this plant as a hair brush. The glue made from this plant was apparently very effective, even in sea water. No one knows exactly how to make this glue anymore.

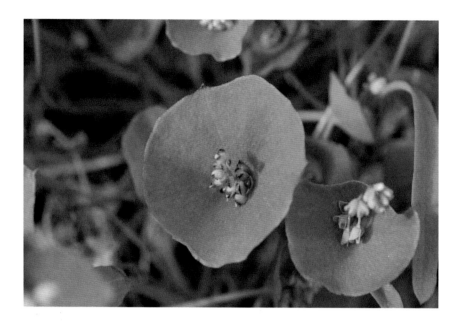

Scientific name – Claytonia perfoliata formerly Montia perfoliata
Common name – miner's lettuce

Identification – This annual plant grows as several kidney shaped leaves that grow on stalks about four inches tall. Each leaf is about three inches wide and entirely surrounds the stalk. Small flowers grow on stalks above the leaves. The flowers are about an eighth of an inch long and are usually white (1).

Characteristics – Miner's lettuce is common in shady, moist areas. It grows in the Spring and is found below about 6,000 feet in elevation (1).

Distribution – The plant is found throughout the Pacific States (2).

Primary uses – The primary use has been and still is as a food (4). The entire plant can be eaten without cooking and tastes like lettuce.

Secondary uses – A tea was made from miner's lettuce and used as a laxative. It was also used as a poultice for arthritis pain (4).

Active compounds – Miner's lettuce has vitamins and minerals and compares favorably in terms of nutrient content with other green, leafy vegetables (70). Claytonia species contain flavonoids such as kempferol and quercetin (71).

Recommendations – Miner's lettuce is a welcome addition to salads and tastes good. It is safe to use, in moderation, a tea made from miner's lettuce as a laxative. It is safe to use miner's lettuce as a poultice for arthritis pain. Discontinue use if a rash forms. People with arthritis should continue to take nonsteroidal anti-inflammatory agents. Miner's lettuce can be grown from seeds available at many nurseries.

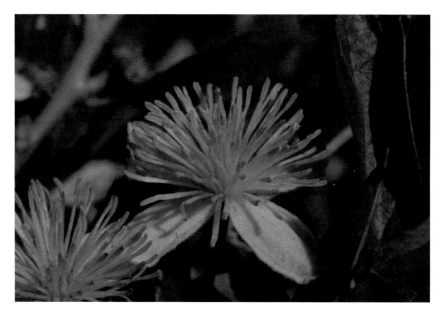

Scientific name – Clematis ligusticifolia
Common name – virgin's bower, yerba de chiva (Spanish), maqshik (pronounced maksheek, Chumash)

Identification – This woody vine can be seen growing on trees and bushes, sometimes high up. The leaves are pinnately divided with five to fifteen leaflets. The leaflets are about two inches long and are irregularly shaped. Actually, they resemble poison oak leaves.

This may disguise the plant, since it often grows on poison oak. The beautiful flowers grow in clusters of many flowers. They have four white sepals that look like petals and are about an inch and a half long. The sepals are hairy on both surfaces. There are many white stamens, about 3/8 of an inch long that are prominent above the sepals. The fruit is made up of many achenes with long feathery styles (1). The Chumash thought the fruit looked like eagle down.

Characteristics – Virgin's bower is fairly common in the Spring and is covered with flowers from April through June. It is found in wet ravines and shady areas below about 7,000 feet in elevation (1). This is probably the plant referred to as coyote's rope in Chumash legends. In these legends, coyote formed his rope into a circle to perform magic, such as finding lost people (72). Coyote stood in the rope circle and prayed in order to find the lost person. The rope was supposed to have been made from plant fibers (such as Apocynum cannabinum) and eagle down. Kawaiisu legends state that grizzly bear used coyote's rope to catch small animals and birds (4). Actually, the vine does not make a good rope, because it is very brittle when dry.

Distribution – This plant is widely distributed. It is found from British Columbia to northwest Mexico and as far east as South Dakota and New Mexico (1).

Primary uses – Virgin's bower was used as a remedy for sore throats and colds (4). The usual method of treatment was to boil the leaves, stems or bark and inhale the steam. However, Indians from Northern California are reported to have chewed the bark and leaves. Chest pains were treated by making a poultice of the leaves and applying that to the chest (4).

Secondary uses – A tea was made from the roots and drunk as an emetic and tonic (4).

Active compounds – Clematis plants contain many triterpenoid saponins (73). These saponins may be sudsing agents that could make soap and shampoo. Some Clematis species have been used to make shampoos. These saponins may also induce vomiting.

Recommendations – The use of virgin's bower as an aromatherapy for colds and sore throats is probably safe. Emetics in general are discouraged because of the danger of inhalation of stomach contents, which can be very dangerous for the lungs. It is not recommended to chew the leaves and bark of virgin's bower due to potential vomiting and other toxicity. The use of virgin's bower as a poultice for chest pains is probably safe, in moderation. Pain in the chest muscles can be caused by over exertion or by excessive coughing. Discontinue if a rash forms, indicating a possible allergy. However, chest pains caused by angina pectoris or heart attack should be treated by a health care provider, without delay. Chest pains caused by tuberculosis or bacterial pneumonia should also be treated by a health care provider. A related plant, Clematis chinensis, is used in China to induce abortions (74). Using any plant to induce abortions is not recommended since in most cases the dose that kills the fetus also kills the mother.

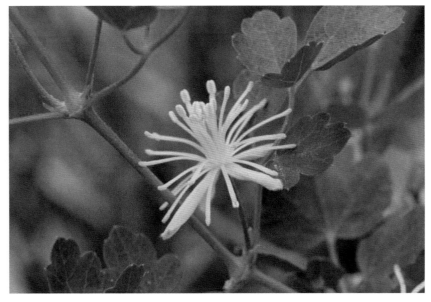

Scientific name – Clematis pauciflora
Common name – ropevine, coyote's rope

Identification – This plant is similar to virgin's bower. It is a woody vine that grows on bushes. The leaves are pinnately divided with three to nine leaflets. The leaflets are about one inch long and are usually three lobed. The flowers look like virgin's bower flowers, but are usually somewhat smaller. They grow in small clusters of one to three flowers. The sepals are hairy only on the underside and are about an inch long. There are many prominent stamens that are about as long as the sepals. The fruit is made up of achenes with long feathery styles (1).

Characteristics – Ropevine is not common and is found in dry chaparral areas below about 4,000 feet in elevation (1). The flowers are usually seen from January to June. Although this plant is called coyote's rope, C. ligusticifolia is probably the coyote's rope from Chumash legends, as discussed under C. ligusticifolia.

Distribution – This plant is found in southwest California and the desert mountains of California (1).

Primary use – The Kumeyaay used this plant to decrease fevers by drinking a tea made from the bark (4).

Active compounds – Ropevine probably contains triterpenoid saponins and other compounds as discussed under C. ligusticifolia. These saponins may cause vomiting.

Recommendations – It may not be safe to drink a tea made from the bark of ropevine. This tea could cause vomiting that is dangerous if stomach contents are inhaled into the lungs. This can result in severe lung damage. Fevers can be safely treated with other plants, such as willow.

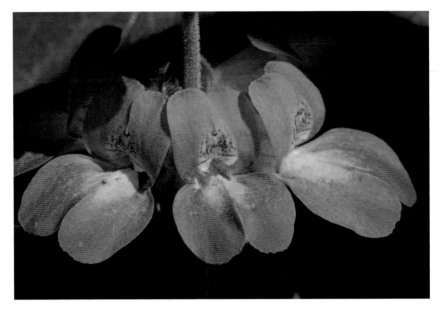

Scientific name – Collinsia heterophylla
Common name – Chinese houses

Identification – This annual plant is usually about a foot tall. The leaves are lanceolate and have teeth on the margins. The flowers have a white upper lip and a purple lower lip (1). They grow in whorls that are supposed to be reminiscent of Chinese houses.

Characteristics – This plant is common and grows in shady places below 3,000 feet in elevation. It blooms from February to May (1).

Distribution – Chinese houses can be found throughout California and northern Baja California (1).

Primary uses – The leaves were used as a poultice for insect or snake bites (4).

Active compounds – There have been no investigations of the active compounds in Chinese houses.

Recommendations – It is not recommended to poultice poison snake bites. Instead, get the victim to the nearest hospital for antivenom treatment. The bites of nonpoisonous snakes should be treated by washing with soap and water then applying a clean bandage. Insect bites should be treated by applying ice for a few minutes to relieve the pain. It is probably safe to apply a poultice of Chinese houses leaves to an insect bite if desired. However, it may be better to leave this beautiful plant for others to enjoy.

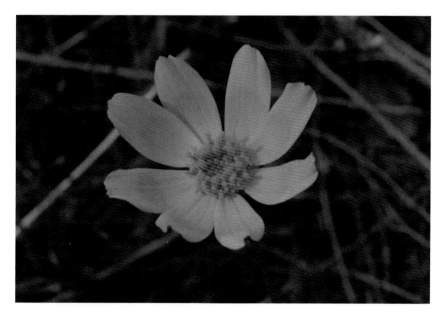

Scientific name – Coreopsis bigelovii
Common name – Tickseed

Identification – This is an annual plant that is low lying. The leaves are pinnately divided into linear segments. The flowers are about two inches wide and form singly on stems about eight inches long. The ligules are yellow, usually darker in the center. The disk flowers, in the center of the flower head, are yellow (1). The flowers form in the early Spring, usually from March to May.

Characteristics – Tickseed is found in grasslands and woodlands bordering the desert. It can be found up to 3,000 feet in elevation (1).

Distribution – This plant is found in central and southern California

(2).

Primary uses – The roots of tickseed were boiled to make a tea that relieved stomach ache, among the Kumeyaay people (4).

Secondary uses – Tickseed was a food plant to many desert people. The leaves and stems were eaten fresh or boiled (4).

Active compounds – Coreopsis species contain many flavonoids, bisabolene derivatives, chalcones and other compounds (75). Phenyl propanoids are present that are anti-inflammatory (76). Some Coreopsis plants are nematocidal (77).

Recommendations – It appears to be safe to eat tickseed. The stems are described as sweet flavored. It is probably safe to use a mild tea made from the roots to treat stomach ache. However, discontinue use if nausea occurs.

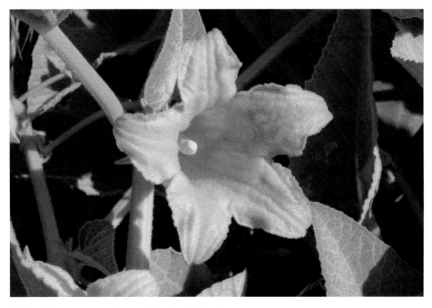

Scientific name – Cucurbita foetidissima
Common name – Calabazilla (Spanish), buffalo gourd

Identification – This ground hugging vine has spiny hairs on the stem. The leaves are ovate, gray-green, covered with hairs and about four inches long. The flowers are yellow, bell shaped and an inch and a half long. The fruit is spherical, green and white striped and about three inches wide (1).

Characteristics – This is a common plant that is usually smelled before it is seen. It has a very acrid, sweat like smell that can be smelled from a distance.

Distribution - It occurs throughout the West in dry, sandy places (1). The fruit is very bitter. This may be one of the plants that zucchini and other squashes are derived from (78).

Primary uses – The flowers were eaten, as were the seeds (4, 27). Salinan people ate the seeds to rid the body of tapeworms (4), which came from eating raw fish, especially freshwater fish. An infusion of the plant was used against gonorrhea and syphilis by Shoshone and Paiute people (79).

Secondary uses – The fruit was used to make soap for washing the body and clothes (4, 78). The roots, which can be large, were eaten to induce vomiting (4). Gourds were used as containers for liquid medicines.

Active compounds – Calabazilla contains cucurbitacins, steroids, triterpenoids, saponins, tannins and organic acids (78). Saponins are detergents and make good soap. Cucurbitacins can be toxic, may be able to inhibit tumor growth and are of interest in cancer research (80). Cucurbita extracts can lower blood sugar and are being investigated by Scientists (81). Extracts of Cucurbita pepo (pumpkin) seeds are used in Europe to treat benign prostatic hypertrophy and acne (3).

Recommendations – It is safe to eat the flowers and seeds. Tapeworms should be treated with drugs known to be effective. Discuss with your health care provider the possibility of adding the seeds to your therapy for tapeworms. Venereal diseases should be treated with drugs known to be efficacious. It is not recommended to use infusions of calabazilla to treat venereal diseases since vomiting may occur. It is safe to use soap made from calabazilla. Do not use the roots to induce vomiting, since vomiting can be dangerous. Inhalation of the stomach contents can cause damage to the lungs. It is safe to use gourds as containers.

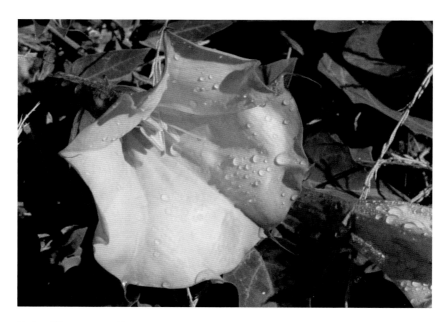

Scientific name – Datura wrightii (formerly Datura meteloides)
Common names – California jimson weed, thorn apple, toloache (Spanish), momoy (Chumash)

Identification – Momoy is a low shrub or vine that can have a repulsive smell, almost like sweat. The leaves are 4 to 6 inches long and are wedge shaped. The fluted flower is about 5 or 6 inches long, and is all white or tinged with purple on the upper edges. The nearly spherical seed capsule is about an inch and a half in diameter, green and covered with spines (1).

Characteristics – The plant is common throughout most of California, except in the desert near Mexico, where a related species, Datura discolor, grows. Flowers appear mostly from July to September, but can be seen at other times as well. The flowers are best seen before the sun rises, when the flowers close. The plant can be perennial or may die out in the winter, depending on the climate. The leaves have a somewhat harsh, astringent flavor.

Distribution – Momoy is found from California to Utah, Texas and Mexico (1).

Primary uses – The root has been used against asthma, nasal congestion and as an anesthetic (4, 15). Broken bones were set using momoy as an anesthetic (4, 15). Many California Indians used momoy root to initiate boys into the religious rites of the tribe. It was the most sacred plant of many California Indian tribes. The plant can induce sacred dreams, hallucinations. Some of the boys died during the initiation due to the toxicity of the plant (15). The initiation was supposed to be a challenge to the boys. According to the Chumash, Momoy was a woman who, as directed by God, created the plant long ago and can be regarded as one of the Chumash Saints (72). Adults have sucked momoy leaves to foretell the future and to prevent damage to their souls by evil (15). If an adult saw a coyote walking like a man, in other words taking human form, this meant the coyote would soon take the adult's soul unless a momoy leaf was sucked.

"Momoy was used to protect the soul. My ancestor, Romaldo worked for an Italian Fisherman (the Italian Fisherman legend #92, reference 72). They went fishing on a small island near Santa Barbara Island. There was a cave on the island where they saw something evil. Romaldo used momoy to protect his soul when he returned home." Frank Lemos (Chumash)

"It has an ability to tickle your soul and bring you back to earth. It brings you into reality. It was what gave you the right to be a man or woman. You were beyond the little girl stage. You wanted to be useful and a part of our community. That was our life." Cecilia Garcia (Chumash)

Secondary uses – Momoy leaves have been applied to bruises and skin irritations to aid healing (4). It has also been used for stomach ache and fever (4). It was used as aromatherapy or as a soaking solution for the feet or head. To make the soaking solution, ferment a small amount of root, or stems, in water for three days, in the sun. Warm the solution on the stove before soaking your feet. The solution can also be rubbed into the scalp.

"I use the stems and crush them for aromatherapy. I have people smell it to awaken the senses, especially people who don't listen well. They need to slow down and open their ears to listen. Other people are oblivious. They don't know how to listen. They're always looking to be offended. With people like that, I say soak your feet. It helps them relax and get their egos out of the way so they can deal directly with God." Cecilia Garcia (Chumash)

Active compounds – Momoy contains scopolamine, hyoscyamine and other active compounds (82). During extraction of the alkaloids in the laboratory, hyoscyamine racemizes to form atropine (S,R-hyoscyamine). These alkaloids are found most abundantly in the young leaves and stems, but are found throughout the plant and seeds. Each seed contains about 0.1 mg of atropine and probably 0.05 mg of scopolamine (83). Poisoning requiring hospitalization can occur eating from as few as 7 seeds. Scopolamine can be very slowly absorbed into the brain in some people, taking up to 13 h to be absorbed. This makes momoy very dangerous since people with slow absorption tend to use more in order to induce the effects. These people tend to use doses that are far too high. The leaves, stems and roots have been reported to contain the same concentrations as the seeds or more of atropine and scopolamine (83). Atropine is used clinically for many conditions including diarrhea, irritable bowel syndrome, hyperactive bladder, asthma, Parkinson's disease and as a preanesthetic agent. Scopolamine has similar uses and is used in motion sickness. Be sure to read the section "Sacred not Psychelic" at the end of the book.

Recommendation – It is safe and advisable to use atropine or scopolamine prescribed by your health care provider, provided you follow your Pharmacist's instructions. This plant should not be used for asthma, since the dose of atropine derived from the plant may vary from plant to plant. It is safer to use medicinal atropine available by prescription. Nasal congestion should be treated with other plants, such as Ephedra viridis, that are safer. Momoy can be used to induce sacred dreams, since this religious practice is protected by religious freedom laws. This is a very dangerous plant. The dose that causes sacred dreams, hallucinations is very nearly the dose that slows down and stops breathing. Only an anesthesiologist should use atropine as a preanesthetic medication, since people can die during anesthesia unless they are carefully monitored. It is safe to apply a momoy leaf to a bruise to aid healing. Discontinue use if a rash forms, indicating a possible allergy. Stomach ache and fever should be treated with drugs known to be effective in these conditions. The presence of atropine and scopolamine in this plant make it potentially dangerous, especially since they can cause fever. It is safe to suck on a small part of a leaf, especially if it protects the soul or helps foretell the future. It is safe to use momoy as aromatherapy, and may help you listen better. It is safe to use momoy to soak your feet, or rub into your scalp, and may help you listen to God. Momoy can be used during religious practices, provided that the dangers of the plant are always remembered.

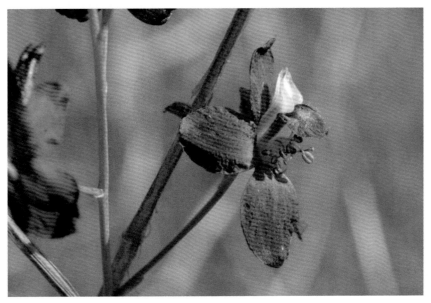

Scientific name – Delphinium parryi
Common name – larkspur

Identification – This plant can grow to be three feet tall, but is usually about eighteen inches. The leaves are curled and covered with very small hairs. The leaves are divided into many, thin lobes. The flowers have five, dark blue sepals that look like petals. The upper sepal has a long spur that is seen on the back of the flower. There are four small petals, that are light blue (1).

Characteristics – Larkspur is common and is found mostly in open woodlands, among grass and in chaparral. It can be found from sea level to 7,000 feet in elevation (1).

Distribution – This plant is found from central California to northern Baja California (1). However, many larkspur species occur throughout the west.

Primary uses – Dried larkspur roots were pounded, mixed with water and used as a salve for swellings (4). It was also used to kill lice, especially head lice (4).

Secondary uses – The leaves and roots of larkspur and other Delphinium species were used as a poison and emetic (4). Stomach aches were commonly treated by emesis. The poison was used against enemies and to make an opponent lose in gambling (4).

Active compounds – Delphinium plants contain many diterpenoids, some of which are toxic, such as methyllycaconitine (84). These compounds inhibit muscle function by inhibiting nicotinic receptors. The inhibition of muscle function leads to cessation of breathing. The compounds are also toxic to the heart causing arrhythmias. Physostigmine is an antidote for the muscle toxicity of larkspur (85). Delphinium diterpenoid alkaloids are under investigation for anticonvulsant effects, narcotic effects, antifungal activity, and antiarrhythmic activity.

Recommendations – It is probably safe to use a salve of larkspur root to treat swellings and lice. The best treatment for swellings is rest, ice, compression and elevation. Larkspur should not be taken internally, since it is very poison. Perhaps in the future, new drugs will be made based on larkspur diterpenoids.

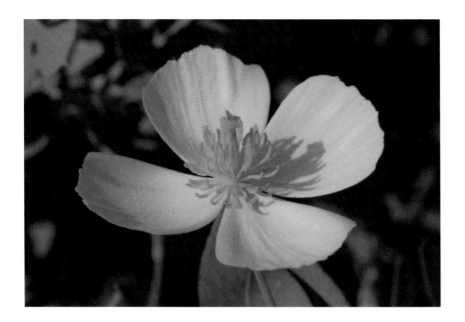

Scientific name – Dendromecon rigida
Common name – tree poppy

Identification – This shrub grows up to nine feet tall. The leaves are elliptic, minutely toothed, about 2 inches long and light green. The poppy like flowers have four satiny, yellow petals and are about an inch and a half wide (1).

Characteristics – Tree poppy is common on dry slopes in the foothills below about 5,000 feet in elevation. It is more common after fires (1).

Distribution – This plant is found throughout California and into northern Baja California (1).

Primary uses – Kawaiisu people mixed tobacco with tree poppy leaves to enhance the strength of the tobacco (4).

Active compounds – There have been no investigations of the active compounds in tree poppy.

Recommendations – Tobacco is highly addictive whether it is smoked or chewed. Smoking tobacco can lead to emphysema, heart disease and lung cancer. It is not recommended to use tobacco except as a ritual herb, where it is burned or given as an offering to God. It is safe to add tree poppy to this ritual tobacco.

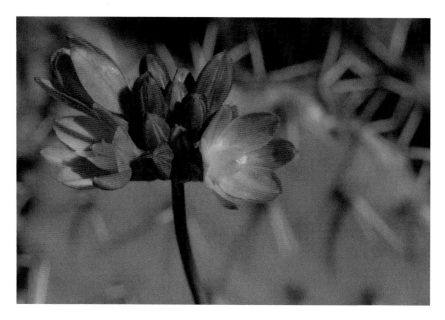

Scientific name – Dichelostoma capitatum
Common name – Blue dicks, cacomites (Spanish)

Identification – This plant grows from a corm and has two or three basal leaves that are about ten inches long. The flowers grow as a head on top of a stalk that is about fifteen inches high. There are two to fifteen flowers that are usually blueish purple. They are bell shaped and about a third of an inch wide. The flowers form in the early Spring from February to April (1).

Characteristics – This is a common plant that is found in woodlands, canyons, chaparral and desert areas. It is a fire following plant and grows abundantly after a fire. It is found up to 7,000 feet in elevation (1).

Distribution – Blue dicks is found from Oregon to northern Mexico and east to Utah and New Mexico (1).

Primary uses – The corms of blue dicks were harvested in large amounts and eaten raw, boiled or cooked in stone lined ovens (4, 69).

Secondary uses – The corms and flowers were used as soap and shampoo (4). Bathing and washing were very important to the California Indians. Soap and shampoo helped them control insect infestations and promoted good skin and scalp health. In the Missions, bathing was not allowed and lead to increased skin, hair and scalp problems (15). The corms were rubbed in a mortar to produce an adhesive (4).

Active compounds – Dichelostoma species contain saponins that are good detergents (86).

Recommendations – It is safe to eat blue dicks, in moderation. Be aware that the presence of saponins in the plants may lead to diarrhea following over eating or insufficient cooking. It is also safe to use the flowers and corms to make soap or shampoo. The corms must be crushed in water to produce a soap or shampoo. The flowers can be rubbed in the hands with water to produce suds. It is safe to make a glue from this plant. The glue was used to seal basketry by the Indians, but could have been useful for holding casts and splints together.

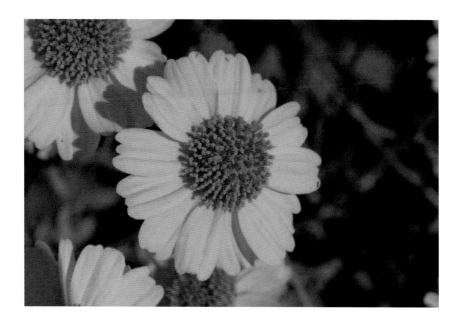

Scientific name – Encelia farinosa
Common name – Brittle bush, incienso (Spanish)

Identification – This bush is usually about four feet tall. The ovate leaves are gray green, covered with matted hairs and about two inches long. The flowers grow on foot long stalks above the bush, have 11 – 21 yellow petals and are brown in the center. The flowers are about an inch and a half wide (1).

Characteristics – This common bush grows in the chaparral, coastal scrub and desert hillsides below about 3,000 feet in elevation (1). It is called incienso because the Spanish sometimes used it as incense in church services (87).

Distribution – This plant is found in Southern California, Nevada, Utah, Arizona and northwest Mexico (1)

Primary uses – The resin from brittle bush was dried into a gum and applied to the chest to relieve chest pain (4).

Secondary uses – The leaves, flowers and stems were made into a decoction, and held in the mouth to treat toothache. A similar decoction was made from Encelia virginensis to use as a wash for arthritis pain (4).

Active compounds – Resin ducts in the leaves and stems produce a resin rich in sesquiterpene lactones, such as encecalin, farinosin, and encelin (88). Sesquiterpene lactones can be toxic, are anti-microbial, insecticidal and can cause rashes (89).

Recommendations – It is probably safe to use the resin from brittle bush externally to treat pain. Discontinue use if a rash forms. Severe chest pain, from angina or heart attack, should be treated in the emergency room by a health care provider. It is not recommended to use a decoction of brittle bush in the mouth. The presence of sesquiterpene lactones may make this decoction dangerous. It is not recommended to use a decoction of Encelia virginensis as a wash since this can cause rashes.

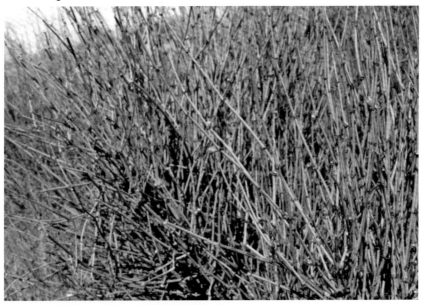

Scientific name – Ephedra californica
Common name – Desert tea

Identification – This plant grows as a shrub, about 4 – 5 feet tall with very few leaves. The stems are yellow-green when young and gray-brown when older. Seeds are found in seed cones that look like very small pine cones, about half an inch long (1). There is virtually no smell to the plant. The taste of the stems is somewhat bitter.

Characteristics – Desert tea is found in many locations, not just the desert. It is found in grassland, chaparral and creosote scrub below about 3,000 feet in elevation (1).

Distribution – This plant is found in Southern California, Western Arizona and Baja California (1).

Primary uses – This plant was widely used as a tea for urinary tract problems, especially when combined with corn silk (4). Corn silk came from the Mohave and Cahuilla people who grew corn (27). It was also widely used to clear up nasal congestion (4). This can be done simply by chewing a stem about the length of the longest finger. Nasal decongestion usually lasts for about an hour and a half.

Secondary uses – The Kumeyaay people used desert tea to treat colds (4). The Kawaiisu used the tea for backaches and as a tonic (4). The dried stems were used as a poultice for sores (4). The Chumash Doctors ('Antap, pronounced gontop) may have used this plant to induce sacred dreams, hallucinations. There are several pictographic depictions of a species of Ephedra, created by the 'Antap. It is widely agreed that hallucinatory plants were used while working the sacred magic of the pictographs (90). The 'Antap claimed do many things, such as cure the sick, by praying and using sacred, hallucinatory plants in front of the proper pictograph.

Active compounds – No California Ephedra species has ever been reported to contain much ephedrine. Ephedrine comes from Chinese, Indian and Pakistani Ephedra species (34). Ephedra californica apparently contains pseudoephedrine, which is a good nasal decongestant and a mild stimulant (91). It may contain other active compounds such as norpseudoephedrine, which is a stimulant and may cause convulsions at high doses (91). Pseudoephedrine can increase heart rate and blood pressure leading to increased urination. This increased urination may be

85

the basis for its use for urinary tract infections. Some Ephedra plants contain quinoline alkaloids that inhibit bacterial growth and may aid in urinary tract infections (92). Pseudoephedrine and norpseudoephedrine are mild stimulants that can induce hallucinations, but only at very high doses. A very large amount of the plant would have to be eaten to induce a sacred dream, hallucination. Eating such a large dose of the plant would be dangerous due to increased blood pressure, that could cause a heart attack or stroke.

Recommendation – Desert tea can be a real aid when hiking with a stuffy nose. Desert tea is a slow growing plant, that should be harvested only in moderation in the wild. If you want to use the plant, buy the plant or the seeds and grow your own. Use it in moderation with the following cautions – hypertension can increase, monoamine oxidase inhibitors can greatly increase blood pressure with pseudoephedrine. In addition, people with hyperthyroidism, diabetes, heart disease, coronary artery disease, increased intraocular pressure, or prostatic hypertrophy should consult their health care provider before using this plant. Pregnant women should not use this plant as discussed under Ephedra viridis. Be aware that this plant is not like Chinese Ephedra, that can be a powerful stimulant and addictive. Desert tea can be used safely in combination with standard antibiotic drugs for the treatment of urinary tract infections. It can also be safely used, in moderation, with standard anti-inflammatory drugs for backache. This plant should not be used as a poultice for open wounds since poultices can contain bacteria and fungi. Wounds should be washed with soap and water and covered with a clean bandage.

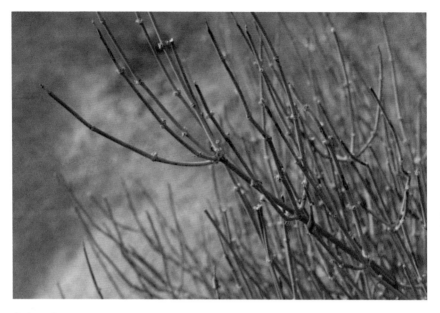

Scientific name – Ephedra nevadensis
Common name – Nevada ephedra, Canutillo (Spanish)

Identification – This shrub grows to about 4 feet tall with a few small, gray leaves, about one quarter inch long. The stems are green and may be covered with powder when young. The seed cones are spherical (1). The plant has very little smell and a somewhat bitter taste, with a juniper aftertaste. This may be the most pleasant tasting Ephedra in California.

Characteristics – Nevada ephedra is found in desert areas of Southern California, especially the Mojave Desert. It is found in creosote scrub and Joshua tree areas below about 2,500 feet in elevation (1).

Distribution – This Ephedra is found in Southern California, Nevada, Oregon and Utah (1).

Primary uses – The Cahuilla used this plant for stomach and kidney problems (4, 27). The Paiute used this plant to treat venereal diseases (29). These diseases may have occurred in California before the arrival of Europeans, but greatly increased in incidence when the Indians were forced to live in Missions (15).

Secondary uses – The stems of this plant and other Ephedras were chewed to alleviate thirst (79).

Active compounds – Nevada ephedra contains little or no ephedrine, but does contain pseudoephedrine (93). Pseudoephedrine can increase heart rate, blood pressure and urination. This ephedra may be the only ephedra species found in California that has substantial stimulant activity. Apparently, norpseudoephedrine, a stimulant, is present in sufficient amounts to cause CNS stimulation. The combination of norpseudoephedrine and pseudoephedrine might increase heart rate and blood pressure enough to be dangerous to some people. Increases in heart rate and blood pressure can lead to heart attack and stroke. Norpseudoephedrine, in very high doses, may also cause seizures. The plant may also contain antibiotic, antimicrobial quinoline alkaloids, as discussed under E. californica. This may be the basis of the use in venereal disease, kidney or urinary problems. The bitter taste of the plant is probably from flavonoids. This bitterness may be the basis of the use for stomach problems and thirst.

Recommendations – This plant in very small amounts, a length of stem less than one quarter the length of a finger, can probably be used safely to alleviate thirst. Bitter plants, such as this, were regarded by California Indians as the best cures for stomach aches. It is not recommended to harvest this slow growing plant in the wild. Seeds and plants can be purchased from nurseries for home use. To use this plant, as with the other Ephedras, make a tea from the stems and use it in moderation. Refer to the cautions listed under Ephedra californica and viridis. Venereal diseases should be treated with drugs known to be effective. Nevada ephedra tea can probably be added safely, in moderation, to this therapy, after discussion with your health care provider.

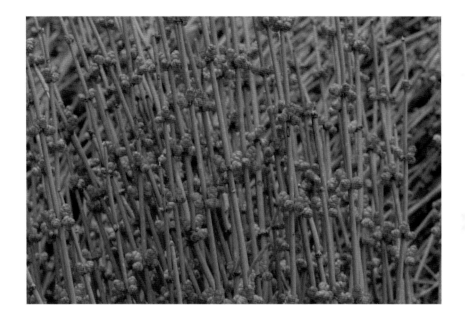

Scientific name – Ephedra viridis
Common name – Green ephedra, joint fir, kiwikiw (pronounced kuwwukka, Chumash)

Identification – This plant grows as a shrub, about 4 – 5 feet tall with a few small, brown leaves about one quarter inch long. The stems are bright green when young and may become yellow with age. The seed cones are more open than with Ephedra californica (1). The plant has very little smell, and a bitter taste.

Characteristics – Green ephedra tends to grow in sagebrush scrub, creosote scrub and pinyon pine juniper woodlands. It grows at slightly higher elevations than Ephedra californica from about 2,000 to nearly 7,000 feet in elevation (1). However, there are several locations where Ephedra viridis and Ephedra californica grow near each other.

Distribution – E. viridis is found throughout the Great Basin all the way to Colorado (1).

Primary uses – A tea was made from the stalks (4) that was used for delayed or difficult menstruation (dysmenorrhea). This plant can also be chewed to clear up nasal congestion. Chewing a length of stem about the length of the longest finger will lead to about an hour and a half of decongestion. Green ephedra was used by the Paiute and Tubatulabal for the treatment of syphilis or gonorrhea (79). These venereal diseases may have been present in California before the arrival of the Spaniards, but increased enormously in incidence in the Missions (15).

Secondary uses – Tea made from this plant was used by many California Indians as a general tonic and against arthritis (79). Green ephedra may have been used to induce sacred dreams, hallucinations by the Chumash Doctors ('Antap, pronounced gontop). The 'Antap created pictographs of this plant. In general, pictographs were used in conjuction with hallucinatory plants in order to perform sacred magic, such as curing diseases.

Active compounds – Ephedra viridis has never been reported to contain much ephedrine. It appears to contain pseudoephedrine and probably norpseudoephedrine (91). The plant is a good nasal decongestant and may be more of a stimulant that Ephedra californica. These stimulant properties may have been the basis for its use as a tonic and against arthritis. Pseudoephedrine clears up the nose by constricting arterioles in the nose. This allows the congestion to drain. Green ephedra may contain antibiotic, antimicrobial quinoline alkaloids that may be useful against venereal diseases, as discussed under E. californica. Both pseudoephedrine and norpseudoephedrine are mild stimulants that could induce hallucinations at very high doses. Such high doses would also induce potentially dangerous high blood pressure leading to heart attack and stroke.

Recommendation – Green ephedra is safe to use for nasal decongestion with the cautions listed under Ephedra californica. The seeds and plants can be purchased for home use. It is safe to use this plant, in moderation, for dysmenorrhea. However, be aware that it can increase blood pressure, which can be dangerous. Dysmenorrhea should be treated with anti-inflammatory drugs. Venereal diseases should be treated with standard drugs known to be effective. However, green ephedra can probably be safely added to standard therapy for venereal diseases, after discussing this with your health care provider. Green ephedra and other Ephedra species have been reported to cause spontaneous abortions (4). It is not clear why it does this. Pseudoephedrine can be used safely, in moderation in pregnancy. However, it is best for pregnant women to avoid any plant that has been reported to cause abortions. Be aware that eating enough of a plant to cause an abortion would almost surely kill the mother as well. It is not recommended to use high doses of this plant to induce sacred dreams since it increases blood pressure and increases the chance of a convulsion or stroke. However, this practice is protected by religious freedom laws.

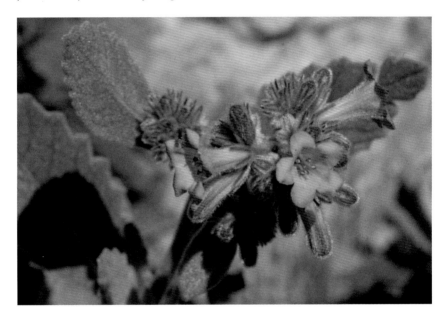

Scientific name – Eriodictyon crassifolium
Common name – Yerba santa (Spanish), wishap (pronounced weeshap, Chumash)

Identification – This shrub can grow to nine feet tall, but is usually about four feet tall. The twigs and leaves are frequently very hairy. The lanceolate leaves are usually about three inches long, with wavy margins or teeth. The flowers are small, less than one quarter of an inch across, lavender and hairy (1).

Characteristics - The plant grows in washes, mesas and ridges up to 7,500 feet in elevation (1). On some ridges, it is the dominant plant. The leaves have little smell but have a sweet, pine flavor.

Distribution – Yerba santa is found in Southern California coastal regions (1). However, a related species, Eriodictyon angustifolium is found from California to Utah and Northern Mexico (1). Eriodictyon californicum is found from California to Oregon (1).

Primary uses – The Chumash used this plant for lung problems including asthma, tuberculosis and pneumonia (4, 15). Bacterial pneumonia was present before the Europeans arrived (15) and was probably a constant concern, especially for children. Before the invention of antiobiotics, bacterial pneumonia contributed greatly to infant and childhood mortality. Tuberculosis may have occurred in California before the Spanish arrived. The incidence of tuberculosis probably increased when the Indians lived at the Missions. Viral pneumonia, especially the flu, seems to have been brought to California by the Spaniards and resulted in many deaths in the Missions (94). The root was chewed or rubbed on the skin to ease aches and pains from arthritis, sometimes called paralysis (4).

"Yerba santa was used for all breathing problems. Hummingbird sage (Salvia spathacea) was used to make yerba santa and other things more palatable because it is sweet. The sticky one (Eriodictyon trichocalyx) tastes better than the fuzzy one (Eriodictyon crassifolium). Yerba santa was sometimes burned for airway problems." Cecilia Garcia (Chumash)

Secondary uses – The leaves of yerba santa were used as bandages, by simply applying a leaf to a cut or scrape (95). The leaves were chewed to increase the flow of saliva and alleviate thirst (95). The Chumash Shamans ('Antap, pronounced gontop) used the plant in a tincture made from eel oil to give power to healing stones (15). Healing stones were usually wrapped in down and placed on or next to a sick person's body to affect a cure.

Active compounds – Plants of the genus Eriodictyon have many flavonoids in them, including eriodictyol, homoeriodictyol, pinocembrin, sakuranetin, cirsimaritin, chrysoeriol, hispidulin, chrysin and others (96). Eriodictyol may have antibacterial, anti-inflammatory and expectorant activities. Eriodicyton californica, a plant found from Southern California to Oregon, was formerly listed in the USA Pharmacopoeia and National Formulary for use in bronchitis but was removed in 1960 when the law required that efficacy had to be demonstrated. No company was interested in paying to conduct the clinical trials to prove the plant was effective.

Recommendations – Asthma, tuberculosis and pneumonia are serious conditions that should be treated with drugs known to be effective. Yerba santa can probably be added, in moderation, to this therapy after discussing the addition with your health care provider. Arthritis should be treated with anti-inflammatory drugs. However, yerba santa can be added safely, in moderation, to arthritis therapy. Yerba santa leaves very quickly stop bleeding of fresh cuts. After the bleeding stops, wash the area with soap and water, and apply a clean bandage. Chewing on yerba santa leaves increases the flow of saliva and is effective at keeping the mouth moist for up to twenty minutes or more. The use of healing stones is no longer understood since the disappearance of the 'Antap.

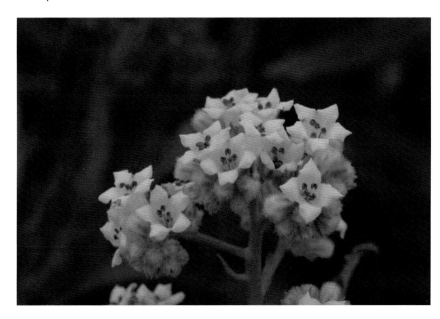

Scientific name – Eriodictyon trichocalyx
Common name – Sticky yerba santa

Identification – E. trichocalyx is smaller than E. crassifolium, growing up to 6 feet tall. The twigs and leaves usually do not have hairs and are covered with a sticky residue. The leaves are lanceolate and about three inches long. They usually do not have teeth and have the margins rolled under. The flowers are less than one quarter of an inch across and are white and lavender or all white (1).

Characteristics - The plant is found in ravines, mesas and ridges up to nearly 9,000 feet in elevation (1). The leaves have very little smell and taste somewhat like pine. The resin from the leaves is persistent and coats the teeth upon chewing.

Distribution – Sticky yerba santa is found in the Southern California coastal and mountain areas, the western edge of the desert and Baja California (1).

Primary uses – Sticky yerba santa was used by the Kumeyaay to treat coughs from any cause (4). The Cahuilla used it for arthritis, tuberculosis, colds and asthma (4, 27). Tuberculosis probably occurred before the arrival of Europeans in California. However, the disease increased dramatically when the Indians were forced to live at the Missions. A tea of the leaves was used for arthritis and lung problems. Usually three leaves were crushed in about half a cup of hot water to make the tea, which was used in small amounts, about a teaspoon at a time. Sugar may have been added. See Carrizo cane for a discussion of sugar.

Secondary uses – The fresh leaves were chewed to moisten a dry, thirsty mouth. A tea was made from the leaves. The leaves were boiled down to make a syrup that was used as candy. A liniment was made from the crushed leaves and rubbed onto sore, tired or arthritic areas. Chewing the leaves was thought to promote the health of gums and teeth (27).

Active compounds – The active compounds in this plant are probably similar to E. crassifolium.

Recommendations – It is safe to chew on sticky yerba santa leaves, in moderation, to alleviate coughs and colds. Tuberculosis and asthma are serious conditions that should be treated with drugs known to be effective. However, sticky yerba santa can probably be added, in moderation, to this therapy. Arthritis should be treated with anti-inflammatory drugs. Sticky yerba santa leaves, teas and liniments can probably be added, in moderation, to this therapy. It is safe to use sticky yerba santa to moisten the mouth. The effect lasts for about 20 minutes. Tooth and gum health is best maintained with a tooth brush. However, chewing on sticky yerba santa leaves, in moderation, would probably be safe for this condition.

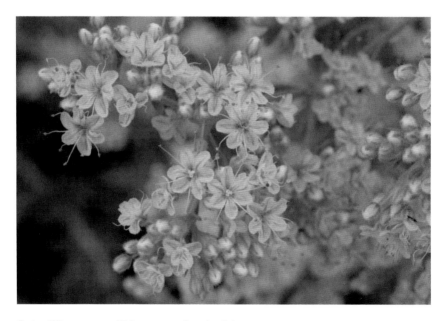

Scientific name – Eriogonum fasciculatum
Common name – California buckwheat

Identification – This shrub is usually about three feet tall. The leaves are oblong and about half an inch long. The flowers grow in an umbel, are pink or white and about an eighth of an inch wide (1). The seeds ripen as the flowers wither to a rust red.

Characteristics – California buckwheat is abundant and is

frequently the most common shrub in the chaparral. It is found in
dry areas below 7,000 feet in elevation (1).

Distribution – This plant grows throughout California and is found
east to Utah and south into Mexico (1).

Primary uses – The seeds of California buckwheat and several
other Eriogonum species were used as food (4, 27). The seeds
can be eaten without preparation, but can also be cooked with
acorns as a soup or bread.

Secondary uses – California buckwheat leaf and stem tea was
used to treat colds, head aches, painful menstruation, urinary tract
infections and back aches. The flowers were used as a laxative,
mouthwash and to treat puss discharges (pyorrhea). A root tea
was used to treat head aches and stomach aches (4, 27).

Active compounds – Very little is known about the active
compounds in this plant or any other Eriogonum.

Recommendations – It is safe to eat California buckwheat seeds.
The taste is coarse and somewhat like saw dust. It is probably
safe to use California buckwheat preparations, in moderation,
for colds, head aches, back aches, stomach aches, as a laxative
and mouth wash. Dysmenorrhea should be treated with anti-
inflammatory agents. It may be safe to add buckwheat to this
therapy. Urinary tract infections should be treated with antibiotics
known to be effective. Puss discharges should be treated with
antibiotics known to be effective.

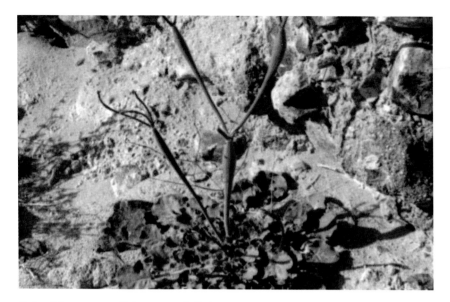

Scientific name – Eriogonum inflatum
Common name – Desert trumpet

Identification – This plant has a hollow stem that is inflated at the ends and the branch points. The stem is green, but fades quickly to brown. The leaves are basal, kidney shaped and about an inch and a half wide. The flowers are yellow, grow in small umbels and are less than an eighth of an inch wide (1).

Characteristics – Desert trumpet is found in the desert in sandy and gravelly areas (1). It is most common near the desert mountains.

Distribution – This plant is found in the desert from California to Colorado and south to Mexico (1).

Primary use – Desert trumpet was used to make smoking pipes. Smoke Doctors used prayer and blew the smoke of burning herbs and tobacco over the bodies of sick people to drive out bad spirits that caused disease (15).

Active compounds – See Eriogonum fasciculatum for a discussion of active compounds.

Recommendations – It is not recommended to inhale the smoke from a pipe. Smoking tobacco damages the airways and can lead to emphysema, heart disease and cancer of the mouth, throat and lungs. Prayer is safe and can be very useful in the treatment of disease. Smoke from burning white sage is frequently used during prayer to take the prayers to God.

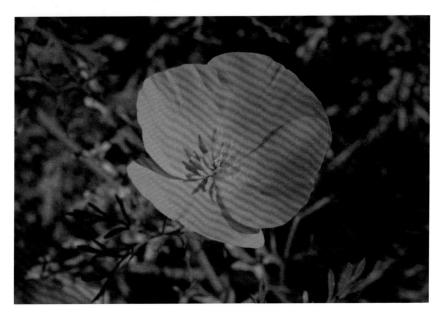

Scientific name – Eschscholzia californica
Common name – California poppy

Identification – This annual plant grows close to the ground. The leaves are basal and are linearly dissected into thin lobes. They have a green or blue green color. The flowers form singly on stalks that are about five inches tall. The flowers are iridescent orange or yellow and about two inches wide. The flowers can also be cream or red colored. They are funnel shaped and have four petals (1).

Characteristics – California poppies are common throughout Southern California and bloom from February to November. They can be found in grassy, open areas up to 6,000 feet in elevation.

They are fire following plants and are much more abundant in the months after a fire (1).

Distribution – California poppy is found throughout California and Oregon (2).

Primary uses – The seeds or seed pods were boiled, mashed and rubbed on the breasts to stop milk production (4).

Secondary uses – The roots were placed in the mouth to relieve tooth ache. See Carrizo cane for a discussion of tooth ache. The root was used to induce sleep. A decoction of the flowers was used to kill lice (4).

Active compounds – There have been no reports of morphine or similar opiate alkaloids in California poppy. The plants do contain several benzophenanthridine alkaloids with antimicrobial activity (97). Extracts of the plant have been found to possess sedative, anxiolytic and analgesic activity (98).

Recommendations – California poppy is protected by law. In order to use the plant, you must grow it in your own yard. It is probably safe to rub California poppy preparations on the breasts to stop milk production. Carefully wash the preparation off the breasts before breastfeeding. Discontinue use if a rash forms on the mother or the baby. It is probably safe to use a decoction of the flowers externally to kill lice. Chewing the root or drinking preparations made from the root should be done with caution and in moderation. Although the leaves of this plant were eaten as greens, this plant is considered to be toxic.

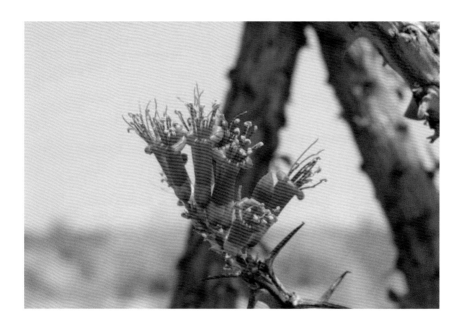

Scientific name – Fouquieria splendens
Common name – Ocotillo (Spanish), candlewood, boojum

Identification – This plant grows to about twenty feet tall or more. Several stems grow from the base and branch only near the ground. Many spines grow from the stems and are about an inch long. The leaves are not usually seen, are spoon shaped and about three quarters of an inch long. The flowers grow in a cyme, have 4-7 petals fused into a tube, are usually red, and about an inch long (1).

Characteristics – Ocotillo is found in the southern deserts (Sonoran) of California. It is found in rocky, dry areas up to 2,000 feet in elevation (1).

Distribution – This plant is found from California to Texas and south into Mexico (1).

Primary uses – The flowers and seeds were eaten. The flowers were soaked in water to make a drink (4, 12).

Secondary uses – The roots were made into a liniment to relieve pains. The roots were made into a tea to treat coughs (4, 12). The bark was used to make gum and wax (99).

Active compounds – Ocotillo contains iridoid glucosides such as splendoside, adoxoside and loganin (100). Iridoid glucosides have antiviral activity and can inhibit the growth of some plants. Also present are eicosane, sitosterol and quercitin (101). Fouquieria species have been used by American Indians to treat cancer (102).

Recommendations – It is probably safe to eat the seeds and flowers of ocotillo, in moderation. It is probably safe to use a liniment made from the roots of ocotillo. Discontinue use if a rash forms. It is probably safe to use a tea made from the roots, in moderation, to treat coughs. It is safe to make gum and wax from the bark. Cancer should be treated with drugs known to be effective, not ocotillo.

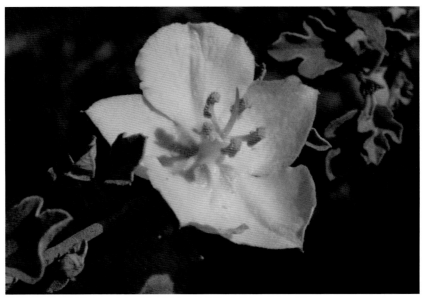

Scientific name – Fremontodendron californicum californicum
Common name – Flannel bush

Identification – This large bush grows to 15 feet tall. The leaves are palmately lobed, an inch and a half wide and feel like flannel. The flowers are two inches wide and have five, ovate, yellow petals. The fruit is an ovoid capsule about an inch wide and covered with bristles (1).

Characteristics – Flannel bush is most common on north facing slopes in the chaparral below about 6,000 feet in elevation. It can also be found in rocky canyons in oak and pine woodlands (1).

Distribution – Flannel bush is found throughout California, Arizona and Baja California (1).

Primary uses – The inner bark was used by the Kawaiisu to relieve sore throats and as a purgative (4).

Secondary uses – The inner bark was used to poultice sores (4).

Active compounds – Nothing is known about the active compounds found in Fremontodendron species. However, the bristles found on the leaves of flannel bush can detach in the skin and cause dermatitis (103).

Recommendations – It is not recommended to use the inner bark of flannel bush internally because vomiting is dangerous. Inhalation of the stomach contents results in severe lung damage and even death. It is probably safe to use the bark to poultice closed sores. Discontinue use if a rash develops. Do not use poultices on open wounds since the poultice can introduce bacteria and fungi into the wound.

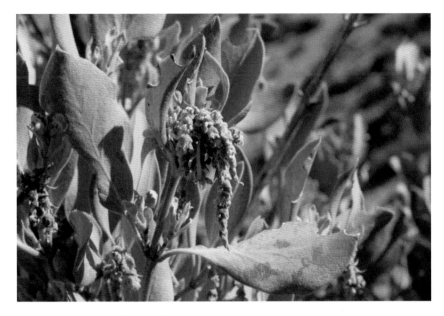

Scientific name – Garrya flavescens
Common name – silk tassel bush

Identification – This bush grows to be 12 feet high. The leaves grow opposite each other on the stem and are longer than wide. The leaves are usually about three inches long and usually have hairs on the underside. The inflorescence is a beautiful pendant catkin-like structure. When freshly formed, the flowers are white and become gray with aging. The round fruit is dark and covered with hairs (1).

Characteristics – Silk tassel bush is uncommon and is found in desert mountains, chaparral and woodlands below 7,000 feet in elevation (1). The flowers form from January to March.

Distribution – This plant is found from California to Utah and south into Mexico (1).

Primary uses – The inner bark was used to reduce fevers (4). Perhaps the inner bark was chewed for this purpose.

Secondary uses – Mojave, Kawaiisu and Kumeyaay people made

the leaves into a tea for stomach aches, diarrhea and colds (4).

Active compounds – There is no evidence that any Garrya
species contains quinine, despite the fact that the bark of the
plant has been called quinine bark. The bark may have been
called quinine bark because of the bitter, quinine like taste. The
bark was used against malaria in California and abandoned when
quinine from Cinchona pubescens became available. Cinchona
pubescens is found on the Amazonian slopes of the Andes from
Columbia to Bolivia. Malaria was introduced in California in 1833,
by trappers from the Hudson's Bay Company (104). Professor
Castillo has estimated that malaria killed 20,000 Yokuts, Chumash
and other interior Indians (105). Malaria remained endemic to
the San Joaquin Valley until 1912 or so, when the large shallow
lakes, Tulare, Buena Vista, Kern and others were drained by
water redirection. The draining of the lakes started in the 1850s,
continued through the 1870s and was completed by the Pine Flat
Dam construction in 1954. These lakes had harbored flocks of
birds numbering in the millions (106). Draining these lakes killed
the huge bird populations that had been characteristic to the San
Joaquin Valley and had supported Indian and condor populations.
It is possible that California condors may not be viable in the wild
until these lakes and bird populations are brought back. Perhaps
Berberis should have been used for malaria. Garrya species
contain several unique diterpene alkaloids such as veatchine,
dihydroveatchine and garryfoline (107). The pseudoindicane
alkaloid, aucubin, may be unique to Garrya (108). Iridoids are
also present including geniposide and geniposidic acid (109).
Flavonoids, coumarins, phenolic acids, lignans, triterpenes and
monoterpenes are also present (108). Some diterpenoids and
triterpenoids are anti-inflammatory agents.

Recommendations – This plant is uncommon and should not
be used for medicine. Willow is much more common and very
useful for reducing fevers and treating stomach aches and colds.
However, silk tassel bush is available from some nurseries.
You can grow this beautiful bush in your own garden and use it
medicinally. It is probably safe to use, in moderation, a tea made
from the inner bark or leaves to treat fevers, stomach aches, colds
and diarrhea.

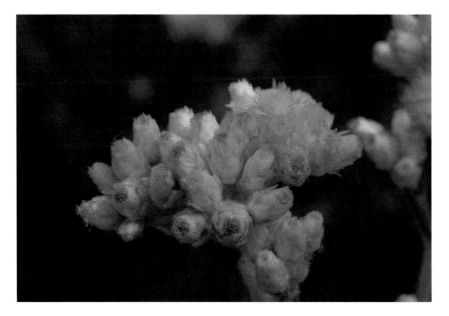

Scientific name – Gnaphalium californicum
Common name – California everlasting

Identification - This plant grows to about two feet tall from a
taproot, is usually branched and can be woolly. The leaves are
lanceolate and sessile. The flowers form in clusters of heads.
Each head is more or less spherical, about a quarter of an inch
wide and white or straw colored. Inside the heads are 50 – 75
very small flowers (1). The flowers smell like maple syrup.

Characteristics – California everlasting can have an orange smell
when the leaves are crushed. It can be seen blooming from
January to June and is found in dry places below 5,500 feet in
elevation (1).

Distribution – This plant is found in California, Oregon and Baja
California (1). There are many species of Gnaphalium that exist
throughout the West.

Primary uses – This plant was used as an analgesic and a
treatment for colds and gastrointestinal problems. It was
apparently used as a leaf decoction (4).

"California everlasting is sweet tobacco, used to change attitudes. I put it over people's eyes, add it to tobacco and have people smoke it, add it to tobacco in water and soak people's feet in it, or use it as a poultice with white sage (Salvia apiana) to pull out bad attitudes that have been held for a long time. I use every aspect of that plant. California everlasting and white sage can be put in a warm, wet towel and used to wrap the heads of cancer chemotherapy patients. Their hair doesn't fall out. They're not in that pitiful state of depression. Let them soak in a tub with it or wrap their heads with it." Cecilia Garcia (Chumash)

Secondary uses – Poultices were made from California everlasting leaves and flowers. The poultices were sometimes applied hot after heating. One Gnaphalium plant, perhaps Gnaphalium stramineum, was reported to enhance female fertility, such that young girls were not allowed near the plant (4).

Active compounds – Gnaphalium plants contain many flavonoids and diterpenes (110, 111). Several of these compounds have antimicrobial activity and may even be effective in pneumonia (112). Some diterpenes are known to have analgesic properties.

Recommendations – It is probably safe to use a leaf decoction of California everlasting, in moderation, for analgesia and the treatment of colds. Poultices for open wounds are not recommended since the plant material can introduce bacteria and fungi. It is best to treat open wounds by washing with soap and water and covering with a clean bandage. It is probably safe to use this plant as a poultice on swollen areas or on the heads of cancer chemotherapy patients. Discontinue use if a rash forms. It is not recommended to smoke anything since this can lead to emphysema, lung damage and other problems. It is safe to use California everlasting as compresses, soaks or poultices to change bad attitudes, especially if it works.

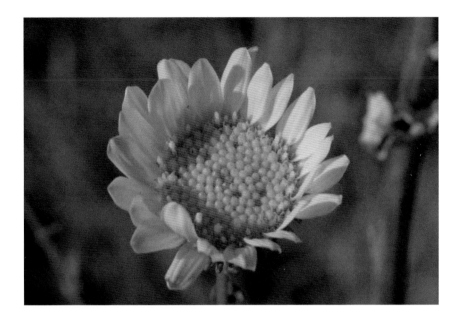

Scientific name – Grindelia camporum
Common name – Gumplant

Identification – Gumplant grows up to one to six feet high. The stems are white or light brown. The leaves are usually an inch long, lanceolate, clasping, entire and gray green. Each stem usually bears one flower of 25-39 ray flowers with ligules about half an inch long. The inner parts of the flower are usually filled with clear gum (1).

Characteristics – This plant is found growing on dry, hot slopes and drainages in full sunlight. It grows below about 2,000 feet in elevation (1).

Distribution – Gumplant can be found from Mendocino to Baja California, and is common in the San Diego area.

Primary uses – Chumash and other people used the plant for asthma, bronchitis, tuberculosis, coughs, sore throats and other respiratory problems (4). Gumplant was also used in US and British hospitals and clinics for the treatment of tuberculosis and other respiratory infections until 1960 (113). In 1960, a US law was passed that required proof of clinical efficacy for all drugs. No company was willing to perform clinical trials with gumplant for fear that a plant preparation could not be patented.

Secondary uses – This useful plant was also used for poison oak rash, skin diseases, lice, as a laxative, for wounds and blood purification.

Active compounds – The plant gum can make up 10% of the plant weight and is rich in grindelane diterpenoids, such as grindelic acid, camporic acid and many others (113). Some of these diterpenoids may have antibiotic effects (113). The plant also contains flavonoids and other compounds (113).

Recommendations – It is safe to use this plant for coughs, sore throats and minor respiratory problems. Consult a health care professional about adding gumplant to bronchitis or asthma therapy. It is safe to use an alcoholic extract of the plant for poison oak rash and minor skin problems. Lice are best treated with louse combs. It is safe to use gumplant in moderation as a laxative. Wounds should be washed with soap and water and covered with a sterile bandage. Blood purification usually involves vomiting, and is not recommended due to the danger of inhaling stomach contents leading to lung damage. Tuberculosis is emerging again as a world problem due to resistance of the mycobacterium. Gumplant and yerba santa have an eighty year history of demonstrated efficacy in US and British clinics against tuberculosis. Gumplant and yerba santa should be examined in clinical trials to see if they are currently useful against tuberculosis.

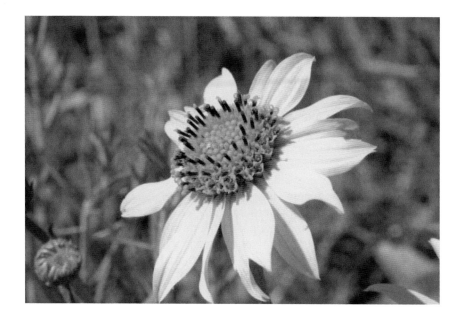

Scientific name – Helianthus gracilentus
Common name – Sunflower

Identification – This sunflower usually grows to about three feet high and has hairy stems. The leaves are opposite, lanceolate and about 4 inches long. The inflorescence is made up of 13-21 ray flowers with yellow ligules about three quarters of an inch long and many disk flowers (1).

Characteristics – This plant if most common after fires and is found on dry slopes in the chaparral below 5,000 feet (1).

Distribution – This sunflower is found from Central California to Baja California (1). There are many Helianthus species that exist throughout the American continent.

Primary uses – The seeds were eaten. Both yellow and purple dyes were made from the plant (4).

Secondary uses – The Shasta used H. cusickii to treat chills and fevers. The root was burned by the Shasta to purify the house after a person died (4).

"The root was used, by the Shasta, to get people unstuck from emotional problems and to help them get over false ideas of what they had to do." Cecilia Garcia (Chumash)

Active compounds – Plants of the genus Helianthus contain sesquiterpene lactones, lectins, flavonoids, benzopyrans, saponins and other compounds (114, 115, 116).

Recommendations – It is safe to eat sunflower seeds and make dyes from the plants. It is probably safe to use the roots, in moderation, against fevers, to purify houses and for emotional problems. Severe emotional problems should be treated by a health care provider who specializes in this area.

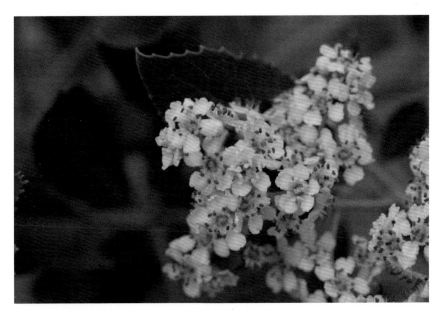

Scientific name – Heteromeles arbutifolia
Common name – Christmas berry, toyon (Spanish), kwe' (pronounce quake, Chumash)

Identification – Toyon grows as a shrub usually about six to ten feet tall. The bark is gray. The leaves are elliptical, evergreen, about four or five inches long and lined with sharp teeth. The flowers grow in panicles in November and December, are white and are about one third of an inch wide. The fruit is shiny, bright red and about one third of an inch in diameter. The fruit forms from November to January. Toyon is found in chaparral, oak forests and evergreen forests below 4,000 feet in elevation. It can grow in wet or dry areas (1).

Characteristics – This is the shrub that gives Hollywood its name. The plant is sometimes called California Holly. Of course very few toyon plants grow in Hollywood now. The berries are edible and have a flavor like a powdery, tart apple. The berries are much better cooked. They can be boiled in a small amount of water to form a sauce that looks like dark red cranberry sauce and tastes somewhat like tart applesauce.

Distribution – This plant is found in California and Baja California (1).

Primary uses – The primary use of this plant was that it was eaten to avoid hunger in the winter time. Winter was the time when people went hungry. The fruit was either toasted with a hot rock in a basket and eaten, or boiled then baked in a pit oven for three days before eating (117). The primary medical use was for women's conditions. Two preparations were used, the flowers were mashed and steeped in hot water or a tea was made from the leaves. These preparations were used to treat irregular menses and probably other conditions (4).

"Toyon berries and elderberries were used to treat senile dementia, now called Alzheimer's Disease." Cecilia Garcia (Chumash)

Secondary uses – A tea made from the bark and leaves was used for aches and pains, including stomach ache. A decoction made from mashed leaves was used to bathe sores. A leaf tea was used as a blood purifier, in other words an emetic (4). The Chumash used the wood of this plant to make bows and hair pins (15).

Active compounds – There have been no reports of the

compounds found in toyon. English holly, Ilex aquifolium, contains a cyanogenic dihydromandelonitrile compound that is responsible for many deaths from eating the plant. However, toyon has been eaten for thousands of years and appears to be safe. The authors have eaten the berries many times, raw and cooked. English holly and California holly are not related plants. They only look like each other.

Recommendations – It is safe to eat toyon berries, in moderation. The cooked berries have a pleasant flavor similar to applesauce and cranberry sauce, especially when sweetened with sugar. As with all plants you have not eaten before, eat it in moderation until you are sure your body tolerates it. It is probably safe to add these berries to the standard therapy for Alzheimer's disease. The use of the leaf tea as a blood purifier or emetic is not recommended. Vomiting can be dangerous and certainly does not purify the blood. Inhalation of stomach contents can seriously damage the lungs. It is not recommended to use a tea of the flowers or leaves for irregular periods or aches and pains. Drinking too much of the tea could lead to vomiting. It is probably safe to bathe sores in a decoction made from the leaves, provided that the area is washed with soap and water afterwards. Washing is necessary to remove any bacteria or fungi that may have been present in the decoction.

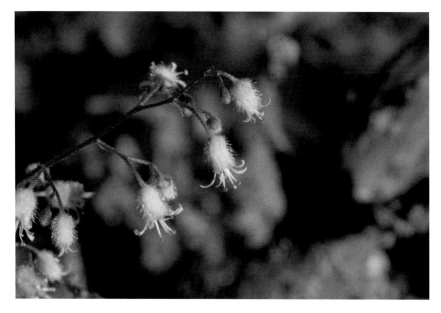

Scientific name – Heuchera rubescens
Common name – Alumroot

Identification – The leaves of this plant are basal and grow on petioles that are up to six inches long. The leaves are broadly ovate and are divided into about seven lobes. They are about five inches in width. The flowers grow as racemes on stalks that are about sixteen inches tall. The flowers have partially fused petals that make a quarter inch long tube and are usually white (1).

Characteristics – This plant is found in dry, rocky areas in the Sierra Nevada Mountains and desert mountains. It grows between 4,500 and 12,000 feet in elevation (1). It is not advised to collect this plant in the wild. There are several Heuchera species and hybrids that can be purchased from nurseries such as Heuchera maxima.

Distribution – This plant grows in California, Oregon, Idaho, Colorado, Texas and Northern Mexico (1).

Primary uses – The fresh roots were eaten to stop diarrhea (4).

Secondary uses – A decoction of the roots were used for many purposes including fevers, heart trouble, liver problems, venereal diseases and as a tonic (4). Liver problems may have been diagnosed by yellowing of the eyes and finger nails. Heart trouble may have been diagnosed as swelling of the feet and trouble breathing at night. Tonics help restore normal blood flow to tissues and may be useful in congestive heart disease.

Active compounds – Heuchera species contain gallotannins that may be responsible for giving the root its bitter and astringent flavor (118).

Recommendations – It is probably safe to use the root of alumroot to stop diarrhea. If diarrhea persists, consult a health care provider. Liver disease, heart disease and venereal diseases are serious illnesses that should be treated by a health care provider. If you want to add a tonic to your heart medicine, discuss it with your health care provider first. Venereal diseases may have occurred in California before the Spanish arrived, but greatly increased at the Missions.

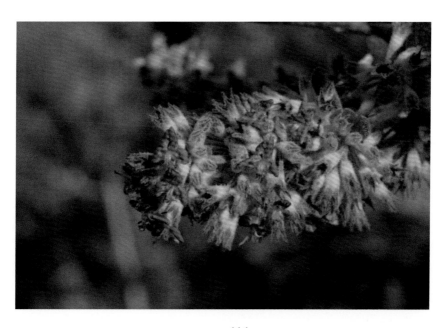

Healing with medicinal plants by Garcia and Adams

Scientific name – Hyptis emoryi
Common name – Desert lavender

Identification – This shrub is usually about four feet tall but can be up to nine feet tall. The branches are hairy when young and become glabrous. The leaves are about an inch long and ovate with a quarter inch long petiole. The small, tubular flowers can be numerous, are purple and are less than a quarter of an inch long (1).

Characteristics – Desert lavender has a fragrant smell, similar to lavender. It blooms in February and March and can be covered with bees. It grows in sandy or gravelly washes and canyons in the desert below 3,000 feet in elevation (1).

Distribution – This plant is found in California, Arizona and Mexico (1).

Primary uses – The flowers and leaves were made into a tea for the treatment of bleeding hemorrhoids and heavy menstruation (4).

Active compounds – Plants of the Hyptis genus are currently of interest for the development of anticancer, anti-AIDS, antifungal, antibacterial, insecticidal and antimalarial agents. There are many active compounds in Hyptis plants including lactones, sesquiterpenes, diterpenes, pectinolides and other compounds (119, 120, 121, 122). Some of the compounds are active against bleeding problems, including hemorrhage caused by snake bites. Other compounds are analgesics. However, the presence of cytotoxic lignans such as podophyllotoxin makes this plant potentially dangerous (123). Podophyllotoxin causes fetal malformations.

Recommendations – This plant should be grown in desert gardens and enjoyed for its fragrance. It should not be used internally, especially not by women of child bearing age, due to the presence of potentially dangerous compounds.

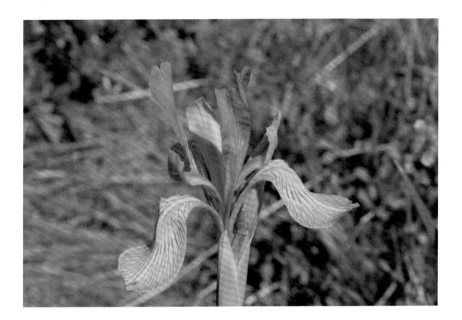

Scientific name – Iris missouriensis
Common name – Western blue flag

Identification – This perennial grows from rhizomes. It grows on a stem that is up to a foot and a half tall. The leaves are up to a foot or more long and a third of an inch wide. The perianth tube, below the flower and above the ovary, is less than half an inch long. The petals have purple and white veins with a central yellow portion (1).

Characteristics – This is the most common iris in Southern California. It is called a noxious weed because cattle will not eat it. The leaves have a bitter taste, to humans. It is found in meadows between 2,500 and 10,000 feet in elevation (1).

Distribution – This plant is found throughout North and Central America (1).

Primary uses – Western blue flag, and perhaps all California irises, were used to make cordage. The cordage was considered very high quality. It is reported that a twelve foot rope of iris requires six weeks to make (4). This cordage may have been used to hold casts and splints together.

Secondary uses – Shoshone people used western blue flag root as an analgesic. For instance, a poultice of the roots was placed on arthritic areas, burns or venereal sores to relieve pain. Venereal diseases may have occurred in California before the Spanish arrived, but greatly increased when the Indians were forced to live at the Missions. A root decoction was drunk for stomach ache and gonorrhea, or dropped in the ear for ear ache (79). Yokuts and Monache people made flour from western blue flag seeds. This flour was used as food (4).

Active compounds – Iris missouriensis roots contains many flavonols, flavones and isoflavones (124). In addition, benzoquinones and triterpenes are present (125, 126). The seeds contain phenols and quinones (127). It is not known which compound in the plant is analgesic.

Recommendations – It is safe to use the fibers of western blue flag to make cordage. It is safe to apply western blue flag preparations externally to control pain. However, if a rash forms, this could be the result of an allergy to the preparation and would preclude further use. It is not recommended to drink decoctions of the roots for gonorrhea, that should be treated with drugs known to be effective. It may be safe to add western blue flag to this therapy after discussing this with your health care provider. It may be safe to use drops of the root decoction for stomach and ear aches, in moderation. The seeds are probably safe to eat, in moderation.

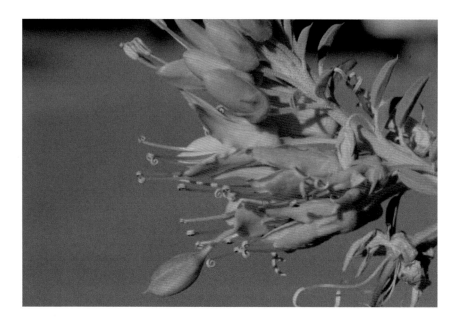

Scientific name – Isomeris arborea
Common names – bladderpod

Identification – This shrub is usually about four feet high and has many branches. The leaves are made of three leaflets that grow at the end of an inch long petiole. The leaflets are elliptical and about an inch and a half long. The showy yellow flowers grow in a long raceme. The petals are about half an inch long and form a bell shaped flower from which the long stamens exert. The fruit are inflated capsules about an inch and a half long (1).

Characteristics – Bladderpod is a common plant that is found on coastal bluffs, in the foothills and in desert canyons. It is found throughout Southern California and can be found up to 4,000 feet in elevation (1).

Distribution – This plant is found in Southern and Baja California (1).

Primary uses – The pods, flowers and seeds were cooked and eaten (4). The young pods have a taste similar to a very mild

118

jalapeno pepper. As the pods age they begin to stink, with a fishy smell. The seeds look like small, brown peas and taste like lentils. However, the Kawaiisu considered the seeds inedible. The flowers and buds were eaten by Tataviam people (129). The flavor is reported to be like a radish.

Active compounds – This plant contains glucocapparin, which gives it a pungent flavor (130). Glucocapparin can be irritating and even causes rashes in some people. Cooking destroys glucocapparin.

Recommendations – This used to be an important food plant that is now entirely neglected. It is being planted in fire sensitive areas, since it does not burn readily. Eating the young pods and the seeds is safe, provided they have been cooked adequately to destroy the glucocapparin. The flavor is pleasant.

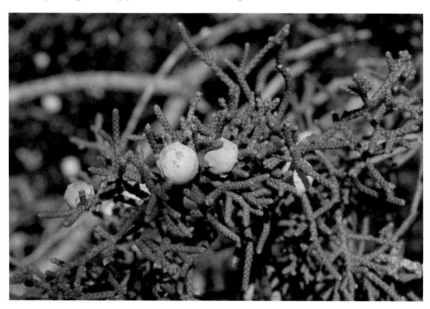

Scientific name – Juniperus californica
Common name – California juniper

Identification – This small tree is usually about fifteen feet tall and has thin gray bark. The leaves are scale like and very small. The pollen cone is less than an eighth of an inch long. The seed cone, also called a berry, is spherical, about half an inch in diameter and purple (1).

Characteristics – California juniper is found most commonly on dry slopes of desert mountains up to 4,500 feet in elevation (1). It can be found growing near pinyon pine trees in some areas.

Distribution – This plant grows in California, Nevada, Arizona and Baja California (1).

Primary uses – The berries were chewed or used as a tea to treat colds and fevers. The bark was used to treat colds, fevers and constipation. The twigs were used to relieve pain and induce sweating. The Kumeyaay made juniper tea to stop hiccups (4).

Secondary uses – The branches were burned to fumigate houses after illness had occurred. The inner bark was used to make diapers and sanitary napkins (4).

Active compounds – Many monoterpenes are present such as pinene, sabinene, limonene and terpinenol (3). Also present are sesquiterpenes, cadinenes, phenols, catechol tannins, flavonoids and leucoanthocyanidins. Berries from Juniperus communis are used to flavor gin and liqueurs and as a spice in food preparation. However, the monoterpenes can be toxic to the kidneys. Overdose makes the urine smell of violets (3). In Europe, a related juniper is used to stimulate the appetite, against heart burn and belching (3).

Recommendations – Juniper must not be used in high doses in urinary tract infections or pregnancy, because of potential toxicity. It is probably safe to use the berries and bark, in moderation, against colds, fevers, hiccups and constipation. Juniper should not be used longer than four weeks at a time. High fevers should be treated with drugs known to relieve fevers. It is probably safe to chew on a small twig to relieve pain and induce sweating. It is safe to use the branches to fumigate areas. It is probably safe to make diapers and sanitary napkins from the inner bark. Discontinue use if a rash forms.

Healing with medicinal plants by Garcia and Adams

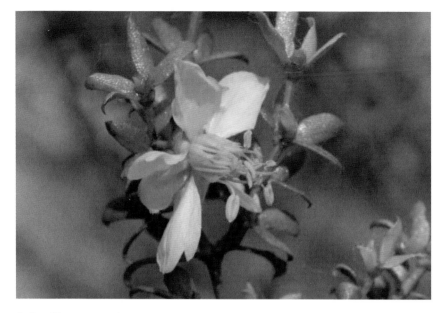

Scientific name – Larrea tridentata
Common name – Creosote bush

Identification – This bush grows to be about ten feet tall. The leaves are made of two leaflets fused at the base. The leaflets are lanceolate, shiny and about a third of an inch long. The flowers have five yellow petals and are about half an inch wide. The fruit is spherical, covered with long, white hairs and less than half an inch wide (1).

Characteristics – This is the most common plant found in many desert areas. It is found up to 3,000 feet in elevation (1).

Distribution – This plant is widespread in the west and is found from California to Utah, Texas and Mexico (1).

Primary uses – The leaves were made into a tea for stomach aches, arthritis pain, colds and menstrual cramps (4).

Secondary uses – The leaves were made into shampoo and poultices (4).

Active compounds – Creosote bush contains phenols, tannins and nordihydroguaiaretic acid (NDGA, 131). The FDA approved NDGA for use in butter and fats to prevent them from becoming rancid. However, FDA approval was removed, in 1968, when NDGA proved to cause kidney and liver toxicity. NDGA was also approved for use against a rare skin disease called actinic keratosis, until it was found that it causes a rash in some people (132).

Recommendations – It may be safe to use creosote bush as a shampoo. Discontinue use if a rash forms. It is not recommended for internal use since using large amounts of creosote bush may cause kidney and liver damage and death. It is not recommended to use creosote bush as a poultice since some people will develop a rash.

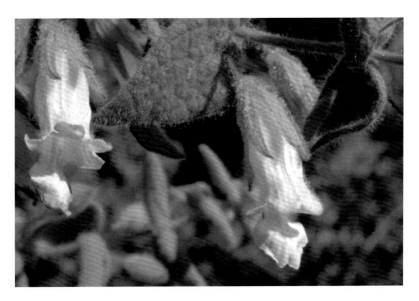

Scientific name – Lepechinia calycina
Common name – pitcher sage

Identification – This shrub has two or three foot long, drooping branches. The leaves are about three inches long and are lanceolate. The branches and leaves are somewhat hairy. The flowers are white and tube shaped with corollas that have five lobes and are about an inch long (1).

Characteristics – Pitcher sage has a very strong, pleasant fragrance that can be smelled from far away. It is mostly found in wooded canyons where it grows in full shade. It is found up to nearly 3,000 feet in elevation (1).

Distribution – This plant occurs throughout California in coastal regions (1).

Primary uses – The leaves were made into a decoction for fever, head ache, the flu and colds (4).

Active compounds – The fragrance of the plant comes from camphor, pinene and similar compounds (133). Many compounds are found in the plant including sesquiterpenes, abietane diterpenes, triterpenes, carnosol, flavonoids, and other compounds (134, 135, 136).

Recommendations – Pitcher sage should be grown in the garden and enjoyed for its pleasant fragrance. Several Lepechinia species have been used in other parts of the world as medicinal plants, especially for uterine infections and diabetes. It is probably safe to use a mild decoction of this plant, in moderation, against colds, flus, and head ache. Serious fevers should be treated with agents known to be effective. It may be safe to add pitcher sage to this.

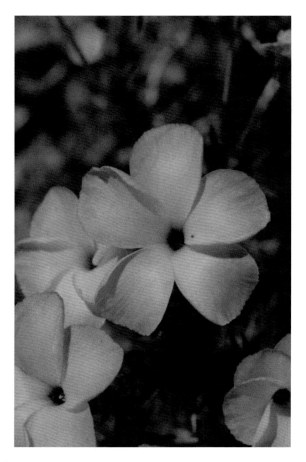

Scientific name – Leptodactylon pungens
Common name – mountain phlox

Identification – This small, perennial shrub grows to about six inches tall. The leaves are divided into linear, spine tipped lobes. The pale pink flowers are open during the day. The flowers are narrow tubes that flute widely at the end. They are about an inch and a quarter wide (1).

Characteristics – Mountain phlox is found is found on some mountain ridges and tops. It is seen throughout Southern California where it grows between 5,000 and 12,000 feet in elevation (1).

Distribution – This plant is found from California to British Columbia and east to the Rocky Mountains (1).

Uses – The leaves and stems of this plant were crushed, mixed with water and used as a bath for swellings, sore eyes and scorpion stings (4).

Active compounds – Plants of the genus Leptodactylon contain a hydroxycoumarin called leptodactylone that is yellow colored (137).

Recommendations – It is probably safe to use a tea made from phlox branches to bath swellings and scorpion bites. The bites of California scorpions are rarely dangerous, but can be painful. Applying ice for a couple of minutes to the bite may help with the pain. It is not recommended to use phlox tea as a bath for eyes. Any preparation placed on the eye must be sterile, or an infection may result.

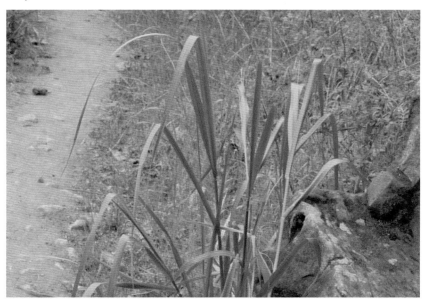

Scientific name – Leymus condensatus
Common name – Carrizo (Spanish), giant rye grass

Identification – This grass grows as clumps of stems that can be up to nine feet tall. The flat leaf blades are about three quarters of an inch wide. A membranous appendage called a ligule is present where the blade and sheath meet. The inflorescence is panicle like, dense and about eight inches long. The spikelets are made up of glumes that are about half an inch long and lemmas that are about a third of an inch long (1).

Characteristics – Before cattle ranchers invaded California, Carrizo was found in the coastal mountain areas growing in huge plains called Carrizo plains. Carrizo grows in open woodlands and canyons below about 4,500 feet in elevation (1). It is a fire following plant and is one of the first plants to grow after a fire. This is the plant that arrow shafts were made from by many California Indians (4, 106). Arrow shafts were made when the shafts were nine feet tall and straightened with hot soapstones.

Distribution – This plant is found from Central California to Mexico (1).

Primary use – Sugar was derived from this cane. Aphids that live on the cane secrete honeydew that is rich in sucrose and many other sugars. The honeydew was collected by thrashing the leaves onto elk hide, dried and formed into balls (106) that looked and tasted like brown sugar. This was one of the sweetening agents of the California Indians. Honey comes from European bees that were imported by the Spanish. There are no California bees that produce honey.

Secondary uses – The Luiseno used a decoction of Carrizo roots as a purgative. It is not safe to use purgatives since inhalation of stomach contents during vomiting can cause lung damage (4).

Active compounds – The sucrose and other sugars in honeydew (138) caused tooth and gum disease among the Indians who collected, traded and ate Chumash candy (also called Yokuts candy). Leymus contains several anthocyanins including peonidin (139).

Recommendations – Honeydew is safe to eat, provided that good dental hygiene is practiced to prevent tooth and gum disease. It is difficult to find Carrizo honeydew these days due to the destruction of the Carrizo plains that used to exist in the coast ranges. The biggest of these plains was 60 miles long and more than 10 miles wide. These plains were a unique ecosystem dominated by Carrizo. Cattle ranching destroyed the Carrizo plains, because cows ate the plant faster than it could grow. Now, giant kangaroo rats, an endangered species, have moved into these areas and preclude the replanting of Carrizo. However, pronghorn antelope, another endangered species in California, are being reintroduced into the Carrizo Plain. Without Carrizo, the antelope will not survive. They need Carrizo to provide cover and protection against coyote predation on their newborns.

Unfortunately, several Anthropologists have mistakenly assumed that Carrizo is Phragmites australis, common cane. Phragmites australis grows near water and never grows to cover huge plains. It was not used to make arrows and is not the source of honeydew that was Chumash candy.

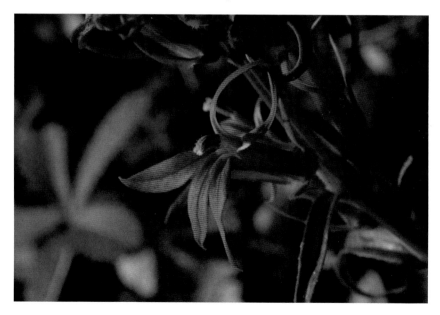

Scientific name – Lobelia cardinalis
Common name – Cardinal flower

Identification – This rare plant grows as erect stalks from one to six feet tall. The stalks can be green or purple-red. The leaves are sessile, lanceolate and about two inches long. The margins are toothed. The large, bright red flowers have two upper lips and three lower lips. The tubes are up to an inch long. The stamens are fused (1).

Characteristics – This plant is becoming more rare every year due to habitat destruction and probably should be called an endangered species in Southern California. It is found growing in or next to streams in full sun. It is found from 1,300 to 5,000 feet in elevation. The open, low elevation streams this plant grows in are virtually gone in Southern California due to redirection of the water for drinking and irrigation. It blooms in September.

Distribution – Lobelia cardinalis is more common in the Eastern US (140). It is found in Texas and Mexico (1).

Primary uses – There are no reported historic uses by California Indians. However, this plant has been very popular among Cherokee and other people, who have moved to California. The Cherokee used it as a poultice for arthritis and other pain. It was drunk as an infusion for respiratory problems. The Iroqois were especially fond of using an external wash made from cardinal flower as a love potion, to help someone find a spouse. The plant was used against syphilis, typhoid, tuberculosis and witch craft (79, 140).

Active compounds – Cardinal flower contains lobeline and other active alkaloids that induce vomiting, stimulate the respiratory system, cause convulsions and death (93). Lobeline was used, unsuccessfully, in smoking cessation programs. It is not addictive. It may also decrease locomotor activity and aggression. Lobeline has some of the actions of nicotine, but is actually pharmacologically different from nicotine (141).

Recommendations – It is not safe to use Lobelia preparations internally due to the vomiting they induce. Vomiting causes death in some people due to inhalation of stomach contents. There have been reports of people trying to use this plant to induce hallucinations. This is very dangerous due to possible vomiting, convulsions and death. It is safe to use cardinal flower as a poultice for arthritis and other pain. It is safe to use a love potion of cardinal flower as an external wash, especially if it works. Discontinue use if a rash forms. Syphilis, typhoid and tuberculosis are dangerous diseases that must be treated by a health care provider. It may be safe to add very small doses of cardinal flower to the treatment for these diseases. A small dose does not cause nausea or other toxicity. It is safe to wear a sachet of cardinal flower against witch craft.

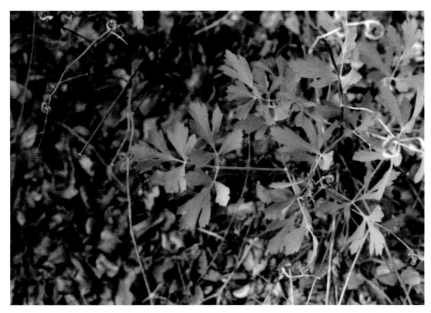

Scientific name – Lomatium californicum
Common names – lomatium, hog fennel, chuchupate (Spanish), chupa' (pronounced chupak, Chumash)

Identification – Lomatium can grow to be about a foot tall. The leaves mostly grow from the base of the plant. The leaves have many leaflets that grow in a wedge shaped, pinnate formation. The tiny, yellow flowers grow in umbels at the top of a foot long stalk. When seeds form, they are prominently visible at the top of the stalk (1).

Characteristics – This small plant grows in woodlands, especially under oak trees, and on brushy slopes in the foothills (1). It usually blooms from April to June, provided there has been enough rain. The seeds are produced soon after blooming. Once the seeds fall off, the plant becomes dormant and will not be seen again until the next spring. The very fibrous, long root smells like celery and tastes like celery.

Distribution – This plant is found in California and Oregon (1). However, there are many species of Lomatium that are found throughout the West.

Primary uses – Lomatium root has been eaten as a treatment for rattlesnake bite. The root may have also been rubbed on the rattlesnake bite. The root was routinely worn on a necklace or belt as a rattlesnake repellant. Chumash Rattlesnake Doctors, in the old days, used lomatium to charm and capture rattlesnakes. The Doctors then danced with the snakes in order to introduce the snakes to the local village people. It was thought that this ceremony would ensure the rattlesnakes would not bite the local people (15).

Secondary uses – The root has been eaten for head ache, stomach problems and arthritis. It was also rubbed on arthritic areas or used as a poultice for sores. A tea made from the root was drunk as a pain reliever. The seeds were eaten for colds, sore throat and other problems. The root, seeds and greens of some species of Lomatium were used as food after boiling (4).

Active compounds – Some species of Lomatium contain suksdorfin and unidentified compounds that have antiviral activity (142). Also present are tetronic acids that are reported to be fish poisons and coumarin glycosides that may affect coagulation (143).

Recommendation – The Chumash claim that lomatium root repells rattlesnakes (15). It is probably safe to wear the root as a rattlesnake repellant, especially if it works. When bitten by a rattlesnake, go to the nearest Emergency Room as soon as possible, to be treated with antivenom. Do not use Lomatium instead of antivenom. Clinical trials and years of experience have shown that antivenom is very effective in the treatment of rattlesnake bite. Lomatium should be investigated in scientific trials to see if it can be used against rattlesnake bite. Lomatium can probably be used safely in addition to standard drugs for arthritis, head ache, stomach problems, sores, colds, and sore throats. Arthritics should not stop taking nonsteroidal antiinflammatory medicines.

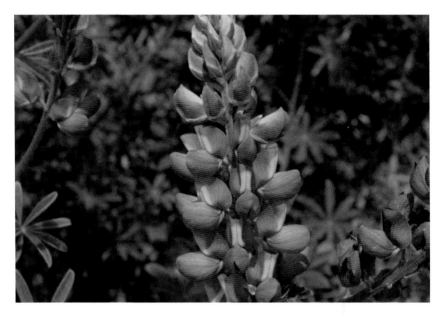

Scientific name – Lupinus excubitus hallii
Common name – Grape soda lupine

Identification – This plant grows about three feet tall and is a perennial. The leaves are up to six inches wide and are palmately divided into about seven usually silver leaflets. The flowers form in long racemes, have keels and lips, and are blue with white banner spots. The fruit are pods that are about two inches long (1).

Characteristics – This plant grows abundantly throughout Southern California in the Spring. It is found below about 9,000 feet in elevation and blooms from February to May. It has a very sweet smell that is reminiscent of the smell of grape soda (1).

Distribution – This plant is found in Southern California (1). However, there are many species of Lupinus that occur throughout the West.

Primary uses – A tea was made from the leaves to treat bladder and urinary tract problems (4).

Secondary uses – Stomach aches were treated by burning Lupinus leaves in the sweat lodge, drinking a leaf tea or mixing the powdered leaves with maple leaf ashes and eating that (4).

Active compounds – Lupinus species contain many alkaloids, including sparteine (144). Sparteine is toxic because it slows down the heart and can cause the heart to stop at high doses (144). This is why California Indians always leached the leaves and seeds of lupine extensively in running water before eating them.

Recommendations – It is not recommended to use arroyo lupine or any other lupine internally due to the potential toxicity of the plant. There are reports of people being hospitalized after eating lupine.

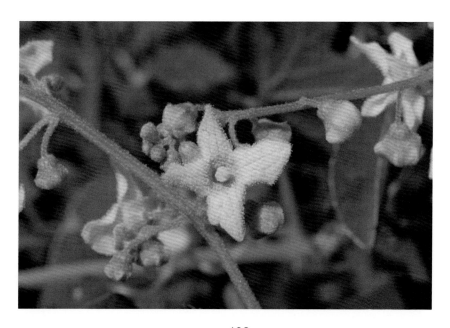

Scientific name – Marah macrocarpus
Common names – wild cucumber, 'anmakhwakay (pronounced ganmakwakkay, Chumash)

Identification – This vine is very common throughout Southern California. It has four inch in diameter, round leaves with five pointed lobes. The stems and leaves are sparsely hairy. The flowers are less than half an inch in diameter and white. The fruit are oblong, green and covered with spines more than an inch long. The fruit are usually about 4 inches long and have four or more oblong seeds about three quarters of an inch long in them. The root of this plant can be very large, hence the name manroot for some Marah species (1).

Characteristics – This plant is found throughout Southern California below about 3,000 feet in elevation (1). The plant is usually the first native plant to bloom in the Spring, with blossoms appearing from January to April. The plant has little smell. The seeds and fruit are extremely bitter.

Distribution – This plant is found in Southern and Baja California (1). However, Marah oreganus is found from California to British Columbia (1).

Primary uses – The seeds were toasted, crushed and used for skin inflammations or stomach ache. The boiled leaves were applied to relieve pain from hemorrhoids and other conditions (4).

Secondary uses – The root was used as a purgative and fish poison. The Tongva used the plant to treat urinary tract problems. An oil pressed from the seeds was used to make pictograph and body pigments. For pictograph pigments, Asclepias sap was added. The seed pods were used to make hair combs. The pods were also used by Shamans to hold poisons. An alcoholic product of the root (or the root of M. horridus) was used to induce sacred dreams, hallucinations and had effects reported to be similar to LSD. The seeds (10 – 15 raw seeds) were used in suicide (4).

Related plants – There are many species of Marah in California. Some of them were used to treat arthritis pain, hair loss, as shampoos, for venereal diseases and other uses (4).

Active compounds – Plants of the Marah genus contain many toxic proteins such as ribosome-inactivating proteins and lectins (145, 146). Many active compounds are found in these plants such as cucurbitacins, pentacyclic triterpenes called maragenins and gibberellin, a plant growth stimulator (147, 148, 149). Some cucurbitacins have antitumor activity. There is a constant need for new anticancer drugs. Perhaps someday, new anticancer drugs will be developed from wild cucumber.

Recommendations – It may be safe to use external preparations of this plant for skin inflammations and pain. If a rash forms, discontinue use since this may indicate an allergy. It is safe to use the oil from the seeds to make pigments. It is safe and advisable to comb the hair, as this can help during flea and louse infestations. The toxicity of this plant makes it potentially dangerous for internal use. The use of purgatives in general is not recommended since inhalation of stomach contents into the lungs is very dangerous. The induction of sacred dreams, hallucinations with this plant is not recommended due to the toxicity of the plant. There is a real danger that hallucinations may be followed by death. However, this practice is protected by religious freedom laws.

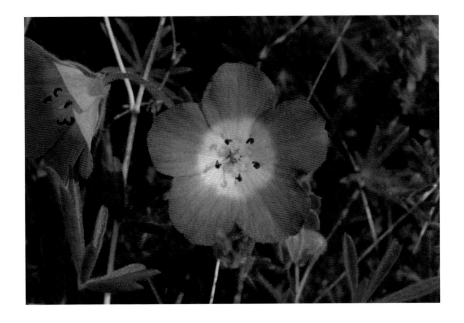

Scientific name – Nemophila menziesii
Common names – Baby blue eyes

Identification – This plant grows as a prostrate or low shrub up to about twelve inches high. The leaves are about three quarters of an inch long, oblong and are pinnately divided. The flowers grow singly from the stem at the leaf petioles. The flowers are bowl shaped and up to an inch and a half wide. There are usually five petals that are blue distally and white medially. Baby blue eyes blooms from March to May (1).

Characteristics – This plant is found throughout California, but seems to be less common than it used to be. It is found in meadows, woodlands and canyons up to 6,000 feet in elevation (1).

Distribution – This plant is found from Oregon to Baja California (1).

Primary use – The root of baby blue eyes was used as a decoction to treat asthma (4).

135

Active compounds – There have been no investigations of the active compounds in this plant.

Recommendations – Asthma should be treated by a health care provider. Talk to your health care provider about adding a decoction of the root of this plant to your asthma treatment. Baby blue eyes seeds can be purchased and grown at home for medicinal use.

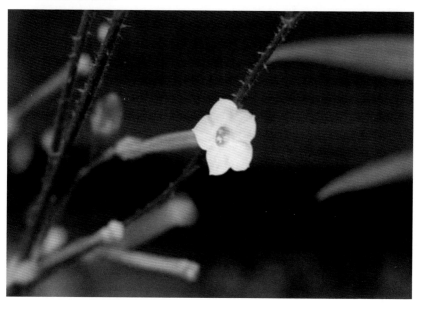

Scientific name – Nicotiana attenuata
Common names – tobacco, pespibata (Spanish), pivat (Cahuilla)

Identification – N. attenuata can grow to be four feet tall, but is usually about two and a half feet tall. The stem is hairy. The leaves are hairy, oblong, about two or three inches long and have a short petiole. The flowers are white, slightly fluted and about an inch and a half long (1).

Characteristics – N. attenuata was one of the four sacred plants of the Mohave and Cahuilla, including corn, squash and beans (4, 27). These plants were carefully cultivated in specially prepared plots. The plants were irrigated either with irrigation ditches or by hand watering (12). The Mohave Indians lived near the Colorado River and used river water to irrigate. The Cahuilla lived in the desert and used spring water from palm oases to irrigate. Every 1 to 4 years, the plots were burned, after the harvest, in order to increase the crop for the next year (27). This plant was also grown by other desert people, such as the Serrano (4). The leaves have a harsh, bitter taste and an unpleasant smell reminiscent of burning rubber.

Distrubition – This plant is found from British Columbia to Montana and south to New Mexico and Northern Mexico (1).

Primary uses – This annual plant and Nicotiana quadrivalvis were used interchangeably to increase alertness and decrease hunger (4, 27). Most California Indians chewed tobacco. However, the Cahuilla smoked tobacco (pivat) in addition to chewing it. Tobacco was the most sacred plant of the Cahuilla. It was given to them by God, Mukat, who created tobacco from his own heart. Tobacco was used to induce sacred dreams, hallucinations by the Cahuilla (4, 27). The Cahuilla apparently habituated themselves to tobacco in order to tolerate the nausea induced by the plant.

Secondary uses – Refer to the discussion for Nicotiana quadrivalvis.

Active compounds – Nicotine is present in this plant, is highly addictive and is discussed under Nicotiana quadrivalvis.

Recommendation – As with Nicotiana quadrivalvis, this is a dangerous plant that should be avoided for induction of hallucinations. The dose required to induce a hallucination is near the dose that causes convulsions and inhibits breathing. However, this practice is protected by religious freedom laws. It can be used safely for external use, as an offering to the fire and for religious uses, provided that the dangers of the plant are always remembered.

Related plant – Nicotiana glauca, also called tree tobacco, is not native to the state of California. The plant was introduced from South America (Bolivia, Paraguay and Argentina, 150) by the Spanish Padres during Mission times. It was used to induce vomiting in order to purge Indians. Nicotiana glauca is a tree about 20 feet tall with large oval, bright green leaves, up to 5 inches long. The flowers are tubular and usually yellow. Nicotiana glauca has been widely embraced by the California Indians since it is easier to grow than the California tobacco plants. The Kumeyaay people call it hutapa erp. Hutapa is coyote in Kumeyaay. Nicotiana glauca contains about 1% nicotine and up to 10% anabasine (150). Anabasine is a compound similar in structure and activity to nicotine, but more toxic in terms of seizure induction. As few as 3 leaves of Nicotiana glauca can be fatal. However, Nicotiana glauca can be used as an effective insecticide against aphids by grinding about 5 leaves in a gallon of water, filtering and spraying the extract. It is recommended that Nicotiana glauca should be avoided except as an insecticide and for use on the skin.

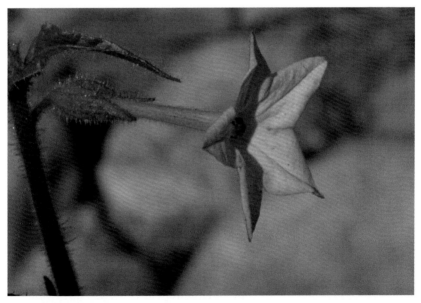

Scientific name – Nicotiana quadrivalvis (formerly Nicotiana bigelovii)
Common names – tobacco, Indian tobacco, pespibata (Spanish), show (Chumash), pivat (Cahuilla)

Identification – N. quadrivalvis can grow to be 6 feet high, but is usually only about 1 or 2 feet high. The stem is hairy. The leaves are oblong, about 2 or 3 inches long and have no petiole. The flower is fluted, white and about two inches long (1).

Characteristics – This annual plant is uncommon and tends to grow in the foothills and where California Indians used to live. This is because many tribes used to plant tobacco wherever they lived and tended it carefully. This involved collecting and sowing the seeds, tending and watering the plants. The flowers appear in May, but can be seen even in October. After harvest, the Chumash and other Indians burned the area every year to increase the crop for the next year (15). The plants can be twice normal size after a fire, with leaves eight inches long and three and a half inches wide. The leaves have a harsh, bitter taste and a pungent, unpleasant smell somewhat like burning rubber.

Distribution – This plant is found from California to Washington and east to the central US (1).

Primary uses – The main uses were to maintain alertness and to decrease hunger pains. Tobacco was especially chewed in the Winter which is the time when people go hungry. The leaves were chewed fresh or dried, sometimes with lime (4). Lime is made by baking clamshells and other seashells in a fire and pounding the baked shells into a powder. Lime is calcium oxide and is a basic compound that can enhance the extraction of nicotine from tobacco.

Secondary uses – Tobacco was used to induce vomiting and as a snuff to clear the head during colds. Many California Indians used the smoke from burning tobacco in a pipe as a means of clearing away evil spirits. Tobacco smoke was frequently used during curing ceremonies. The Doctor blew smoke over the body of the sick person in order to drive out the evil spirit that was the cause of the sickness. The smoke was also blown into a person's ear to cure ear ache. Tobacco leaves were used as poultices for cuts, bruises, wounds and on the neck for tuberculosis and sore throat. For arthritis, tobacco leaves were placed on hot rocks in the sweat house. The patient breathed the steam from the tobacco leaves to alleviate arthritis. There are reports of California Indians using tobacco to induce sacred dreams, hallucinations (4, 15).

"Tobacco is used for prayers as an offering of strength. It is also smoked as a deterrent for pests, ticks, flies and other things. Infections are pulled out by tobacco, open sores or thoughts."
Cecilia Garcia (Chumash)

Active compounds – Nicotine in tobacco (151) is very addictive and is a stimulant. It causes tremors and at higher doses, convulsions that can be fatal. Nicotine initially stimulates breathing and at higher doses inhibits breathing. Vomiting is a prominent effect of nicotine (152).

Recommendations – This is a dangerous and addictive plant that should be avoided. There are better ways to stay awake, such as with coffee. Nicotine induced hallucinations are dangerous because the dose required is very close to the dose that inhibits breathing and causes convulsions. However, this practice is protected by religious freedom laws. These hallucinations are accompanied by profuse vomiting. Purging by vomiting is not recommended in general, because inhalation into the lungs of the vomit can be life threatening. Using tobacco smoke to drive away evil spirits is recommended, if it works. However, breathing tobacco smoke is bad for health and can lead to emphysema, heart disease and cancer. Use of poultices is safe only as a temporary measure until a clean bandage can be applied. Poultices can contain bacteria and fungi. All cuts and wounds should be washed with soap and water. Ear infections should be treated with antibiotic drugs. Tuberculosis may have occurred in California before the Europeans arrived, but was an uncommon disease until the Indians were forced to live in Missions. Tuberculosis is a very serious condition that should be treated with drugs known to be effective. However, wearing tobacco leaves around the neck is safe, even in tuberculosis and sore throat. Aroma therapy with tobacco leaves for arthritis is probably safe, provided that standard arthritis drugs are also used. It is safe to use tobacco as an offering of strength during prayer. It is safe to soak in preparations of tobacco in water to pull out infected thoughts.

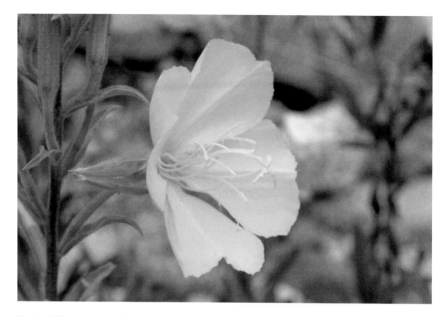

Scientific name – Oenothera elata
Common name – Evening primrose

Identification – This is a large, short lived plant that can grow to seven feet tall. The leaves are about four inches long and are lanceolate. The yellow flowers are about three inches across and have four petals that are notched. The stigma rises above the stamens. The fruit is a narrow cylinder about two inches long (1).

Characteristics – This is a common plant in Southern California and is planted in many gardens. It grows in moist places below about 5,000 feet in elevation (1).

Distribution – This plant is found throughout the western US and Central America (1).

Primary uses – "Evening primrose helps women stay balanced and helps their dreams." Cecilia Garcia (Chumash). A leaf tea or flower tea was used to help with yeast infections, urinary tract infections, pregnancy or menopause. The tea helped the woman adjust to the changes of pregnancy and menopause.

"When you look at today or a thousand years ago, a woman is the foundation of society. She cannot afford to be wounded by disease." Cecilia Garcia (Chumash)

Active compounds – Evening primrose contains flavonoids, tannins, gallic acids, fatty acids, sterols and other compounds (153, 4). Gallic acid is active against fungal infections (153). Extracts of evening primrose can also decrease cholesterol levels and inhibit coagulation (155, 156).

Recommendations – It is safe and soothing to drink primrose tea. Urinary tract infections and yeast infections can be treated, in part, by drinking fluids such as the tea. The presence of gallic acid and similar compounds in the tea may make it useful in the treatment of urinary tract infections and yeast infections. However, these infections can be dangerous and should be treated with agents known to be effective. Evening primrose tea can probably be added, in moderation, to this therapy. The reported ability of evening primrose extracts to lower blood cholesterol levels could make this plant very useful in menopausal women whose cholesterol levels may increase. Talk to your health care provider about adding this tea to your cholesterol lowering medication.

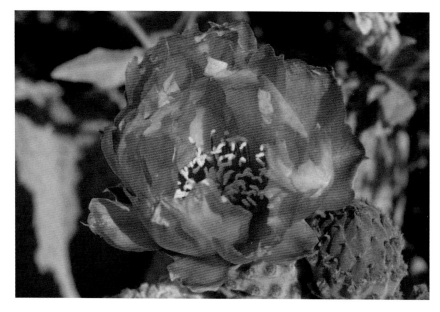

Scientific name – Opuntia basilaris
Common name – Beavertail cactus

Identification – This cactus is usually found growing in small clumps of three or four feet in diameter and up to about two feet tall. The segments are flat and grow in the shape of a beaver tail. The segments have few spines, but many bristles. The bristles can penetrate the skin even though they are small. The flowers are about four inches wide with dark pink perianths, that look like petals, and magenta filaments. The fruit is green and purple and dries out to tan (1).

Characteristics – Beavertail cactus is found in the desert, chaparral and up to the juniper pinyon pine woodlands. It grows in very dry, sunny areas up to 6,500 feet in elevation (1).

Distribution – This cactus is found from California to Utah and south into Mexico (1).

Primary uses – This cactus was used as food, as described under O. littoralis.

Secondary uses – After removal of the spines from the pads, wounds were dressed with the pads as a poultice and a pain reliever (4). Shoshone people rubbed the bristles into warts and moles to remove them (140).

Active compounds – Refer to O. littoralis.

Recommendations – It is safe to use the pads and fruit of beavertail cactus for food. The fruit can be eaten raw or boiled. The pads should be boiled and fried before eating. Be sure to remove all bristles before eating. The pads can be used as a poultice for the relief of pain. Dressing wounds with this poultice should only be a temporary measure until the wound can be washed with soap and water and a clean bandage applied. Poultices can contain bacteria and fungi. It is not recommended to remove warts or moles with the bristles of beavertail cactus. This could result in infection.

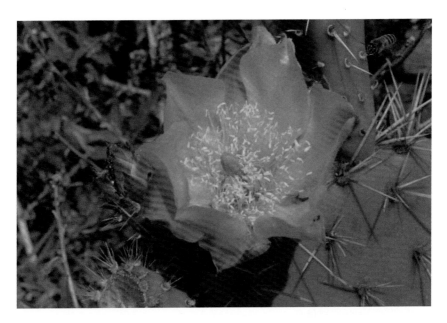

Scientific name – Opuntia littoralis
Common name – prickly pear cactus, kwukwu (the u is pronounced as in cup, Chumash)

Identification – This cactus grows in clumps of up to twenty five feet in diameter and perhaps eight feet tall. The cactus grows in flat, elliptical segments with many spines. There are four to eleven spines in each areole with the longest spines reaching an inch and a half long. The flowers are about four inches wide and are usually yellow but can be red (1). The fruit (tuna in Spanish) is red or purple, full of round seeds and can be very sweet with a taste reminiscent of guava. Be careful when removing the spines from the fruit.

Characteristics - This is probably the most common Opuntia cactus in Southern California. However, it hybridizes readily with most other Opuntia species, making identification impossible in some locations. It is found in coastal sage areas and inland chaparral up to 1,200 feet in elevation. It can grow in wet or dry areas (1). Perhaps the best tasting fruit prickly pear fruit is found on Catalina Island.

Distribution – This cactus is found in Southern California and Mexico (1).

Primary uses – Perhaps all Opuntia species were used as food, even the jumping cholla that is so full of spines. The pads and fruit were used as food. The fruit was occasionally boiled into a sauce that was allowed to ferment into an alcoholic beverage before drinking (4).

Secondary uses – Prickly pear was used as a poultice for wounds. The spines were removed. The pads were split and applied to the wound. They were also applied to ease swelling and the pain of bites, or arthritis (4). Prickly pear was frequently planted near villages in order to have food nearby. It also may have served as a prickly fence.

Active compounds – The pulp from some species of Opuntia can contain large amounts of glucose and fructose, some vitamin C, 5% protein, some starch, pectin and other constituents (157). Opuntia plants contain beta-sitosterol and perhaps other anti-inflammatory agents (158). Extracts of the stems of some species have been shown to promote wound healing and to be analgesic

(159). The pads (nopales in Spanish) have been shown to decrease the blood levels of glucose, total cholesterol and LDL-cholesterol (160, 161). Extracts of a species of Opuntia have been found to have antiviral activity (162).

Recommendations – It is safe and highly recommended to eat the fruit of prickly pear cactus, provided that the spines have been carefully removed. The fruit can be eaten raw or boiled. The pads should be boiled, then fried before eating. A temporary poultice can be made from the pads. However, the time required to remove the spines before applying the poultice precludes using it as an emergency measure. Poultices can contain bacteria and fungi and should only be used temporarily. Wash all wounds with soap and water before applying a clean bandage. It is safe to use the pad as a poultice for pain and swelling. Bites, especially animal bites, should be treated by a health care provider. It is safe to use this plant as a fence, provided that children are warned about the spines. Hopefully in the future, preparations of prickly pear cactus will be available for use in wound healing, inflammation relief and analgesia. It is safe and recommended to eat the pads of this plant to help control blood glucose and cholesterol. Please discuss this use with your health care provider.

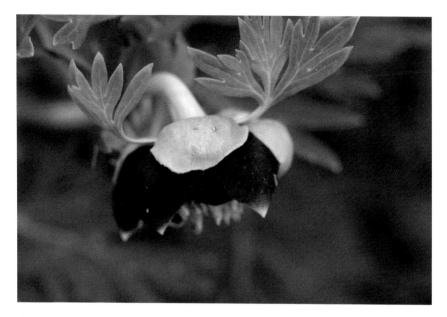

Scientific name – Paeonia californica
Common names – California peony, mim (pronounced meem, Chumash)

Identification – This subshrub grows with many branched stems from the root base. The plant can be nearly three feet tall. The leaves are deeply cleft into compound formations and are generally four or five inches wide. They are dark green above and paler below. The flowers are large, about four inches wide, have dark red petals and prominent yellow filaments and anthers. The fruit forms as large, green follicles up to an inch and a half long. Three follicles form from each flower (1).

Characteristics – California peony is most common in coastal scrub and chaparral near the coast, especially two or three years after a fire. It can also be found in moist ravines in the foothills. It is found from about 500 to 4,500 feet in elevation (1). It blooms early in the Spring, usually in February and March.

Distribution – This plant is found in Southern California (1). P. brownii is found from Northern California to British Columbia and east to Wyoming (1).

Primary uses – The tuber of this plant was made into a tea and used to treat depression and lung infections such as from colds (4). The tea was also used to treat neuralgia, which is pain radiating along a nerve (16).

Secondary uses – The tuber tea was used to treat menstrual cramps, stomach ache, head ache, as a laxative, for urinary tract problems, poison oak rash, and as an emetic (4, 15).

Active compounds – Major constituents of peony tuber include penta-O-galloyl-beta-glucose, paeoniflorin and paeonol (163, 164). Tuber extracts contain antioxidants, such as suffruticosides and galloyl-oxypaeoniflorin, that are more powerful radical scavengers than vitamin E (165). Paeonimetabolin-I and similar compounds are anticonvulsants (166). Paeonilide, a monoterpenoid metabolite, and two acetophenone derivatives from peony are anticoagulants (167, 168). Paeoniflorin can increase blood pressure (169). Blood sugar levels decrease following paeoniflorin or 8-debenzoylpaeoniflorin administration (170). Peonans, acidic polysaccharides from peony tuber, can stimulate the immune system (171). An extract of Chinese peony tuber can stimulate the recovery of fibrotic liver (172). Chinese peony extracts can lower blood cholesterol and partially prevent atherosclerosis (173). Chinese peony extracts can also improve heart function in heart disease (174).

Herbalist uses of peony – Peony plant extracts are used for many conditions especially in Europe and China. European and Chinese peony tuber extracts are used for many conditions ranging from arthritis to epilepsy. Clinical trials of peony in Germany have found that it is not useful and not recommended for any condition (3). Peony is still the most popular herbal medicine in China.

Recommendations – It is probably safe to use, in moderation, a tea made from the tubers of California peony for colds, stomach ache, and as a laxative. Depression is a serious condition that should be treated by a health care provider. Neuralgia, such as from shingles, can probably be safely treated with peony tuber tea, in moderation. In general, it is not safe to use emetics since inhalation of stomach contents can result in serious damage to the lungs. Menstrual cramps and head aches should be treated with anti-inflammatory drugs, perhaps in combination with peony. Urinary tract problems should be treated by a health care provider. However, a tea made from peony tubers may be helpful in stimulating urination. It is probably safe to bathe poison oak rash in a lukewarm peony tuber tea. Discontinue use if the rash gets worse, since this could be due to an allergy to peony.

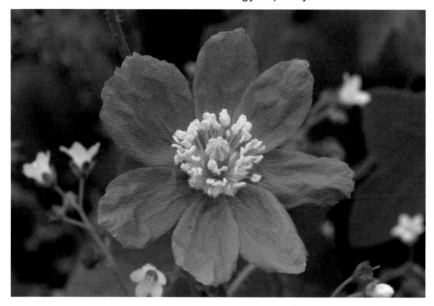

Scientific name – Papaver californicum
Common name – Fire poppy

Identification – This annual grows to one or two feet tall and is sometimes very hairy. The leaves are pinnately divided and are about two inches long. The flowers have four or more brick red or orange petals, each with a white spot at the base and are about an inch and a half long. The seed pod is about half an inch long (1).

Characteristics – This plant grows only during the year or two after a fire and only in certain areas. There are apparently three major requirements for growth of fire poppies, a fire, adequate rainfall, and a coastal California location. The plant is found below about 2,400 feet in elevation. Fire poppies are not cultivated because no one has figured out how to grow them from seeds. The Chumash, however, grew fire poppies in their fields.

Distribution – Fire poppies are found only along the Central and Southern California coast (1).

Primary uses – The only information available about fire poppies comes from Chumash legends. For instance, the gates of heaven, Similaqsa, are guarded by two huge ravens, qaq. The raven's eyes are like mirrors that force the soul to examine itself to find if it is truly worthy to enter Similaqsa. If a soul is worthy to enter into heaven, the ravens pluck out the soul's eyes and replace them with poppies (72).

Active compounds – There have been no investigations of the active compounds in fire poppies. However, opium, morphine, heroin, codeine and other compounds are produced from the latex of the opium poppy, Papaver somniferum. The seed pods of fire poppies are small compared to opium poppies and produce very small amounts of latex.

Recommendations – Fire poppies are very rare. Less than 50 specimens were reported in 2004, and fewer than that in 2003. They should not be gathered or used at all. Hopefully, someday they will be cultivated and we will learn more about them.

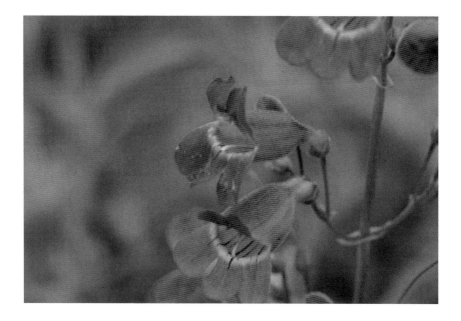

Scientific name – Penstemon spectabilis
Common name – Royal penstemon

Identification – This plant is usually about three feet tall. The leaves are lanceolate and fused at the bases, surrounding the stem. They are folded lengthwise and have teeth along the margins. The flowers are purple and have a long corolla tube with five calyx lobes. They are about an inch long (1).

Characteristics – Royal penstemon is found in gravelly and sandy soils along washes, in coastal scrub, in chaparral and oak woodlands. It generally blooms in March and April. It grows up to 7,000 feet in elevation (1).

Distribution – This plant is found in the mountains near Los Angeles and south to Baja California (2). However, there are many closely related penstemons found throughout the West.

Primary uses – Many penstemon species were used as poultices to treat sores, swollen limbs and skin disorders (4).

Secondary uses – Other penstemons were used to treat kidney disorders and to comfort people suffering from grief (4).

Active compounds – Penstemon species contain iridoid glycosides, phenylpropanoid glycosides, alkaloids and other compounds (175). The biological activities of these compounds are of interest to Scientists and include: wound healing, anti-inflammatory, antimicrobial, immunostimulant, antiviral, antiplatelett and many other activities (176). Many of these activities would be beneficial in poultices.

Recommendations – It is probably safe to use penstemon in poultices of sores and swollen areas. Discontinue use if a rash forms. It is not recommended to use on open wounds or sores due to the possibility of introducing bacteria from the plant. Kidney diseases should be diagnosed and treated by a health care provider. Discuss the possibility of using penstemon to treat grief with your health care provider.

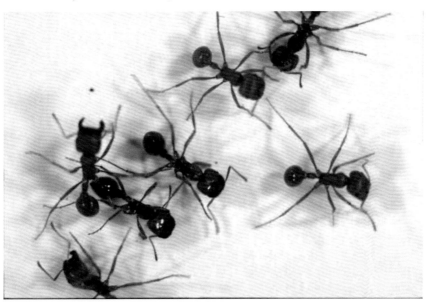

photograph by Robert Roberts

Scientific name – Pogonomyrmex californicus
Common names – red harvester ants, shutulhul (pronounced

shuetulhul, Chumash)

Identification – This is an ant, not a plant. But it has been a very important and useful medicine for a long time. Harvester ants are small, about a half inch long or less. They are red brown in color and can be identified by the fact that they are usually seen carrying seeds and other plant materials. They are usually active in the morning and evening. Their nests are usually surrounded by mounds, up to 3 or 4 inches high, and 2 to 4 feet wide, of plant detritus.

Characteristics – Harvester ants live in the foothills in large mounds. These ants are being threatened by Argentine ants that have invaded California. The small, combative Argentine ants can easily wipe out harvester ant colonies.

Distribution – Harvester ants are found mostly in the coastal areas of California.

Primary uses – These ants have been used as a potent cure for diarrhea, even the diarrhea associated with dysentery (15). The ants were administered by an ant Doctor, usually a woman. About 200 – 450 live ants were consumed in each treatment. The Doctor scooped up the ants on eagle down, then popped the ants and down into the mouth of the patient, who was instructed to swallow quickly. Of course, the ants stung the inside of the throat and mouth as they were consumed.

Secondary uses – Eating the ants can induce hallucinations. Some Chumash boys were initiated into the religious rites of the tribe by eating ants in order to experience a sacred dream, hallucination. This was considered safer than using Datura wrightii (15).

Active compounds – The exoskeleton of ants is made of chitin and chitosan that have antibiotic activity (177). The ant stings introduce formic acid and other irritants that can damage tissue and red blood cells. The sting venom contains polypeptides called kinins that have a number of activities (178). Kinins cause pain, inflammation, and can lower blood pressure. The kinins in ant venom may be able to induce hallucinations due to their activities in the brain. It could also be that the seeds harvested by the ants are sometimes infected with Claviceps fungi that produce ergot alkaloids, that are hallucinogenic. Ants may eat Claviceps fungi and concentrate ergot alkaloids in their bodies, although this is not currently known.

Recommendation – It is not recommended to eat live harvester ants. Fried ants or other ant preparations should be active against diarrhea, and should be much safer than eating live ants. Several scientific investigations have shown that it is safe and effective to use insect chitin or chitosan in the treatment of diarrhea. There is a constant need for new antibiotics and antiprotozoal agents, especially new compounds that work by new mechanisms. Be aware that giardiasis and other protozoal infections of the guts can be very serious conditions that should be treated with drugs known to be effective. It is not recommended to eat live ants in order to induce hallucinations. This is a potentially dangerous activity that could kill as easily as inducing a hallucination. There are no records of the cause of death from eating ants. However, this is an established religious practice that is protected by religious freedom laws. If ants are used for religious purposes, please be aware of the potential dangers.

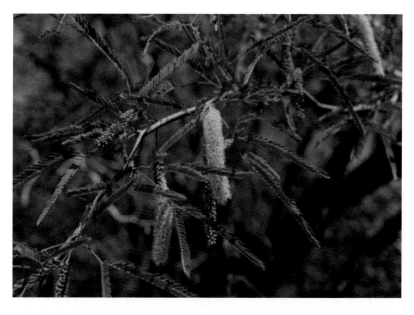

Scientific name – Prosopis glandulosa
Common name – honey mesquite, ah pee (Paiute)

Identification – This large tree can grow 20 feet tall and spreads with many stems to become 50 feet wide or more. The leaves are pinnately divided into 7-17 pairs of opposite leaflets. The leaflets are oblong and about half an inch long. Spines occur in pairs on the smaller branches. The tiny, yellow flowers grow in hanging spikes that are about two and a half inches long. The fruit are tan pods that are about five inches long. Inside is a soft brown pulp and several flat, oblong seeds. The seeds are about a quarter of an inch long (1).

Characteristics – Honey mesquite is common in desert areas of the San Joaquin Valley and Southern California. It occurs in grasslands, canyons and mesas up to 5,000 feet in elevation (1).

Distribution – This plant is found in the San Joaquin Valley and Southern California (1).

Primary uses – Honey mesquite provided food and shelter. The pods were eaten and have a very pleasant, sweet taste. The spreading trees were used as homes, with rooms created under and between the lower branches (12.

Secondary uses – The leaves were boiled to make a tea for diarrhea, head aches, sore throats and stomach aches (4, 12). The sap was boiled to make glue. A mixture of the sap and mud was used to remove lice from the hair (4).

Active compounds – Prosopis plants contain many flavonoids, tannins and ellagic acid (179-181). However, it is the abundance of alkaloids that is of concern to cattle, sheep and goat ranchers. When animals eat diets high in mesquite, they develop brain damage that can be fatal (182, 183). It is not known which alkaloid damages the brain. Many alkaloids are present such as prosopinine, tryptamine, eleagnine, harman, catechin and phenethylamine.

Recommendations – Honey mesquite pods have been eaten for centuries by the desert people of California. It is probably safe

155

to eat these pods, in moderation. It is safe to seek shade under a honey mesquite tree, provided that the thorns are avoided. It is not recommended to use the leaves to make teas due to the possible presence of alkaloids that could be dangerous if consumed in large amounts. It is safe to use the sap to make glue or to remove lice. Discontinue use if a rash forms.

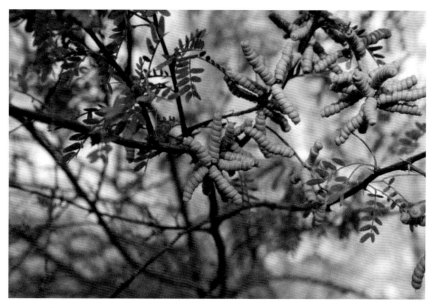

Scientific name – Prosopis pubescens
Common name – screwbean mesquite, tornillo (Spanish), quier (Paiute), qwinyal (Cahuilla)

Identification – This tree can grow to 30 feet tall and tends to occur in groups. The leaves are pinnately divided into 5-8 pairs of opposite leaflets. The leaflets may be hairy, oblong and are about one third of an inch long. Spines occur either singly or in pairs on the smaller branches. The tiny flowers grow in pendant spikes about two inches long. The fruit are brown pods that grow tightly coiled in a spiral structure and are about two inches long. Inside the pods are very small, black, spherical seeds and a soft, dark brown pulp (1).

Characteristics – Screwbean mesquite is uncommon in California and is found in sandy washes in the desert. It can be found up to 4,000 feet in elevation (1).

Distribution – This plant is found from the deserts of Southern California to Texas and Northern Mexico (1).

Primary uses – The pods of screwbean mesquite were used as food (4, 27) and have a very pleasant, sweet taste.

Secondary uses – The roots and bark were used as medicines by the Cahuilla for unidentified purposes (27). They may have used them similarly to the Pima of Arizona (79). Screwbean roots were used, by the Pima, as a decoction or powdered and applied to sores and wounds. A root infusion was used, by the Pima, for menstrual problems. The pods were used to make a fermented drink by the Mojave people.

Active compounds – See Prosopis glandulosa for a discussion of the active compounds.

Recommendations – It is probably safe to eat the pods of screwbean mesquite, in moderation. It is probably safe to drink a fermented, alcoholic drink made from the pods of screwbean mesquite. It is not recommended to drink more than one alcoholic drink a day due to possible damage to the body caused by long term use of alcohol. It is not recommended to use a root or bark preparation of screwbean mesquite internally due to the possible presence of potentially dangerous alkaloids.

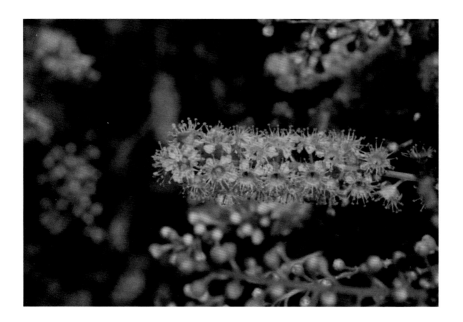

Scientific name – Prunus ilicifolia ilicifolia
Common names – Holly leafed cherry, islay (Spanish),
'akhtatapush (pronounced gaktattappush, Chumash)

Identification – This plant is usually a shrub about 15 feet tall, but
can be a tree up to 30 feet tall. The leaves are evergreen with
petioles a third of an inch long. The leaves are round and lined
with spines. The flowers grow in dense racemes. The flowers are
white and about a quarter of an inch wide. The fruit is spherical,
about three quarters of an inch in diameter and is green, red or
purple. There is one large stone in the fruit (1). The pulp forms a
thin layer over the stone and tastes like a cherry, but not as sweet.

Characteristics – Holly leafed cherry is found in canyons,
shrubland and woodlands below about 5,000 feet in elevation (1).
It usually grows in the shade of trees or boulders. Holly leafed
cherry and redberry frequently grow side by side and are difficult
to distinguish until the fruit forms. The fruit forms in July and
August.

Distribution – This plant grows from Northern California to Baja California (1).

Primary uses – The pulp was eaten fresh off the plant. The stones were cracked open to extract the kernels. The kernels were leached with water before they were cooked and mashed into something similar to the consistency of refried beans. The kernels have a mild, sweet flavor. These kernels were almost as important as acorns as a food (4).

Secondary uses – A tea was made from the bark to treat colds. The steam from boiling leaves was inhaled to relieve the flu. A leaf decoction was used as a wash for head aches (4).

Active compounds – The leaves, roots and flowers of Prunus species contain flavonoids, triterpenes, sterols, anthocyanins and several antioxidant compounds (184-186). The leaves of Prunus species also contain prunasin, that releases cyanide (187). This can lead to cyanide toxicity when leaves are eaten. The fruit of Prunus species is rich in sugars, fiber, minerals and antioxidants (188). The kernels of Prunus ilicifolia appear to contain amygdalin, that releases cyanide (187). This is why the Indians leached the kernels with water and cooked them extensively into a mush before eating them. This process avoided cyanide toxicity.

Recommendations – It is safe to eat the kernels of holly leafed cherry provided that the ancient technique is followed for preparation and cooking. This involves chopping the kernels, leaching in running water for several hours and extensive cooking to produce a mush. Improper preparation and cooking may lead to cyanide toxicity. It is not recommended to use internal preparations of the bark or leaves, due to the possible presence of prunasin that can cause cyanide toxicity. It is not recommended to inhale the steam from boiling the leaves since cyanide can be released into the steam. It is probably safe to use a leaf decoction as an external wash for head aches. Discontinue use if a rash forms.

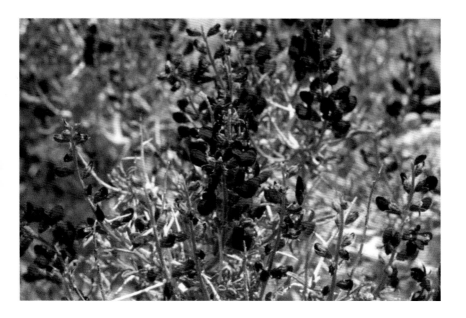

Scientific name – Psorothamnus fremontii
Common name – Fremont's indigo bush

Identification – This low bush is usually about eighteen inches to three feet tall. The branches are silver colored. The leaves are pinnately divided into three or five leaflets about a quarter of an inch long. The flowers occur in racemes, are purple with red bases and look like pea flowers. They are less than half an inch long. The seed pod is about one half of an inch long and is a capsule with lines of small reddish brown glands. The glands make the seed pods look like they are covered in caramel.

Characteristics – Fremont's indigo bush is rare in California and found in the desert mountains of the Mojave Desert, especially the Grapevine Mountains. It grows in sandy washes, volcanic slopes and canyons up to 4,000 feet in elevation. The plant blooms in June. The leaves smell like mild sage and taste like grass. This plant looks very similar to Psorothamnus aborescens. The two species can be distinguished only by the seed pods and were probably used similarly.

Distribution – In California, this plant is only known with certainty in the Grapevine, Providence and Whipple Mountains near the California border with Nevada. It is more common in Nevada and Utah (1).

Primary uses – The roots or leaves were used to stop internal hemorrhages. The roots were made into a decoction for stomach aches (79).

Active compounds – Psorothamnus species contain isoflavones such as fremonin and fremontone (189). Also present are heterocyclic compounds such as psorothamnone, dalrubone and emorydone (190). Some of these compounds are being investigated for anticancer activity.

Recommendations – This plant is very rare in California and is a slow growing plant that should not be harvested in the wild. If it is growing on your property, you can use it. Internal hemorrhages should be treated in the Emergency Room of a hospital without delay. It is probably safe to treat stomach aches, in moderation, with a root decoction of this plant.

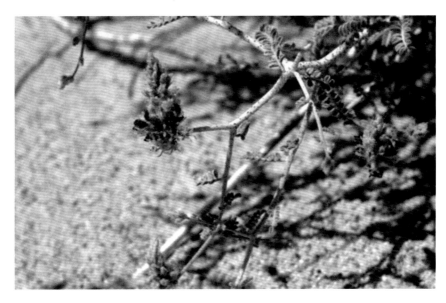

Scientific name – Psorothamnus polydenius
Common name – Nevada smokebush

Identification – This spreading shrub grows to about four feet tall. The twigs have many orange-yellow glands. The leaves are pinnately divided into 7-13 leaflets that are about an eighth of an inch long. The flowers form in densely hairy spikes, are pink-purple and look like pea flowers. They are less than a quarter of an inch long (1).

Characteristics – This plant is most abundant in sand dune areas of the eastern Mojave Desert, especially the Eureka Dunes. It grows between 2,500 and 6,500 feet in elevation. It blooms in May (1).

Distribution – This plant is found in the deserts of California, Nevada and Utah (1).

Primary uses – The Paiutes and Shoshone used this plant for many purposes. The stems were chewed to relieve pain and to treat colds and flus. An infusion of the plant was used against diarrhea. A decoction of the stems and leaves was used to stimulate urination and treat urinary tract disorders (79).

Secondary uses – A decoction of the leaves and stems was used as a wash for measles and small pox. The plant was used for venereal diseases and tuberculosis (79). Small pox was brought to California by Europeans (94). Venereal diseases and tuberculosis may have occurred in California before the Spanish arrived, and increased greatly at the Missions.

Active compounds – See Psorothamnus fremontii for a discussion of active compounds.

Recommendations – This is a slow growing desert plant that should not be harvested in the wild. You can use it if it is growing on your property. It is probably safe to use Nevada smokebush for pains, colds and flus. Mild diarrhea can be treated, in moderation, with Nevada smokebush. If diarrhea persists for more than two days, it should be treated with preparations known to be effective. Urinary tract infections should be treated with antibiotics known to be effective. It is probably safe to wash the skin of measles patients with a decoction from this plant. Small pox is extinct. Venereal diseases and tuberculosis should be treated with drugs known to be effective. Discuss with your health care provider adding Nevada smokebrush to your standard drug therapy.

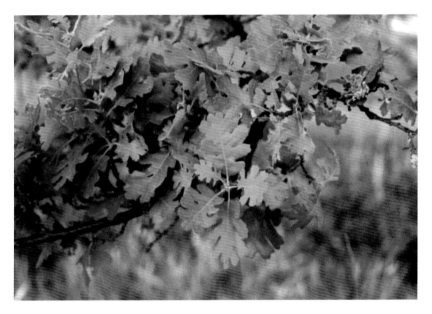

Scientific name – Quercus lobata
Common name – Valley oak, roble (Spanish), ko (pronounced koe, Chumash)

Identification – This is a very large tree that grows to one hundred feet tall. The oblong leaves are about three inches long with a quarter inch long petiole and deeply divided into 6-10 lobes. The acorns are about an inch wide and up to two and a half inches long (1).

Characteristics – This once common tree is now becoming very uncommon in Southern California as trees are cut down and habitat is destroyed. This is the favorite acorn producer of most Indians and was probably planted by them wherever they lived. It grows in oak woodlands below about 5,000 feet in elevation (1). It is a slow growing tree such that a tree with a three foot trunk radius is probably about 350 years old or so.

Primary use – Acorns were the most important food during the winter (4). Acorns were collected in the Fall and stored for up to four months in granaries. Acorns are susceptible to mold, weevils and dessication. Acorns were eaten as a porridge, soup or baked bread by many Indians. The Kumeyaay and others ate acorns as a cold pudding.

Secondary use – A thin acorn soup was administered as the first therapy for almost any disease, especially diarrhea, among the Chumash and other Indians (15). An infusion of powdered oak bark was used externally for skin problems, arthritis pain and burns. This infusion or a leaf decoction was used internally for colds, stomach aches, child birth and as a poison (4).

Active compounds – Acorns are about 6% protein, 20% fat and 65% carbohydrate (4). They provide good nutrition and taste good when properly prepared. Cattle may die from eating whole acorns or oak leaves due to phenolic compounds that can cause liver and kidney damage (191). These phenolics and tannins are removed by washing with baking soda and water. Deer routinely eat acorns. Oak contains monoterpenes, flavonoids, and many types of gallates and tannins (192-4). These tannins are important in the wine industry, since wine is frequently aged in oak barrels.

Recommendation – . It is probably safe to use bark or leaf preparations on the skin. Discontinue use if a rash forms. It is not safe to use bark or leaf preparations internally due to possible liver and kidney damage by phenolic compounds.

Acorns should be eaten as follows. Place the meat of about 40 acorns in a blender. Fill half full with water and add a teaspoon of baking soda. Process for about 30 seconds and allow to settle for 10 minutes. Pour off the liquid and wash by processing with fresh water, twice. Pour the acorns into a bowl and cook in the microwave oven for about 5 minutes, until the acorns are chocolate brown. Eat this porridge with brown sugar for an authentic California Indian taste. Thin with hot water to make the thin acorn soup. To make a somewhat bitter pudding, refrigerate the processed acorns, do not cook them.

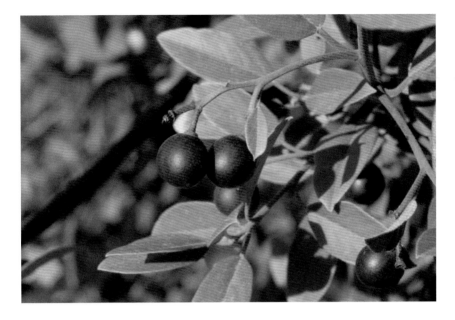

Scientific name – Rhamnus californica
Common name – Coffeeberry

Identification – This large shrub can grow to fifteen feet tall. The bark is gray-brown. The leaves are evergreen, elliptic and about two and a half inches long. The petioles are almost half an inch long. The very small, white flowers grow in small umbels. The berries are about half an inch in diameter and are red or black (1).

Characteristics – Coffeeberry grows in coastal scrub, chaparral and forests up to 7,000 feet in elevation (1). It usually grows under the shade of trees. The berries have a mildly bitter flavor.

Distribution – This plant is found in California and Southern Oregon (1).

Primary uses – The bark and berries were used to induce vomiting and as a laxative (4).

Secondary uses – The sap and leaves were used against skin rashes, wounds, burns, infections and warts. The bark was used against mania, urinary tract problems and arthritis pain (4).

Active compounds – Rhamnus species contain many flavonoids, naphthalene glycosides and anthraquinone glycosides (195-197). Some of the flavonoids have anti-inflammatory and anticoagulant activity (198, 199). The Anthraquinone glycosides are laxatives and emetics (200). They exert their action by damaging the cells that line the gut.

Recommendations – This plant has been used for centuries by Indians and the Spanish as a laxative. It is probably safe to use coffeeberry, in small amounts, as a laxative. It should be used only occasionally, not long term. The chronic use of anthraquinone agents may lead to gut damage. Using coffeeberry to induce vomiting is not recommended since vomiting can be dangerous, if the stomach contents are inhaled into the lungs. It is not recommended to use coffeeberry to poultice open wounds since this can introduce bacteria and fungi into the wound. It is probably safe to use coffeeberry preparations on closed sores, burns and arthritic pains. Discontinue use if a rash forms. Mania and urinary tract infections should be treated with drugs known to be effective. It may be safe to add coffeeberry to standard therapy for these conditions after discussion with your healthcare provider.

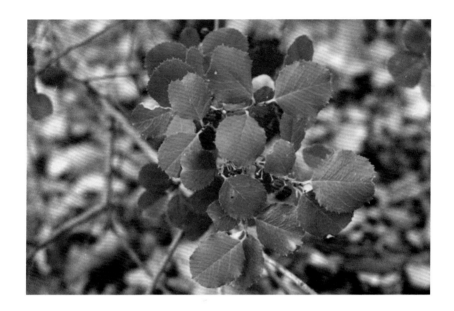

Scientific name – Rhamnus ilicifolia
Common name – Redberry

Identification – This shrub grows to about twelve feet tall. The bark is gray. The evergreen leaves are about three quarters of an inch long, round and have many spines along the edges. The very small, white flowers grow in groups of about six and have no petals. The berries are about a quarter of an inch long, have two stones and are bright red (1).

Characteristics – Redberry grows in the chaparral and forests up to 6,000 feet in elevation (1). It is usually found growing in the shade of trees. The berries have a sweet and bitter flavor and form in June and July.

Distribution – This plant is found in California, Arizona and Baja California (1).

Primary uses – The roots and bark were used for laxative effects (4).

Secondary uses – The roots and bark were used against colds, pains, to increase urination, stomach aches and skin swellings (4).

Active compounds – See coffeeberry for a discussion of the active compounds in Rhamnus species.

Recommendations – It is probably safe to use redberry for occasional constipation. However, long term use is not recommended since gut damage may occur. It is probably safe to use redberry, in moderation, for occasional pain, stomach aches, skin swellings and to increase urination. Colds can probably be safely treated with redberry on a short term basis.

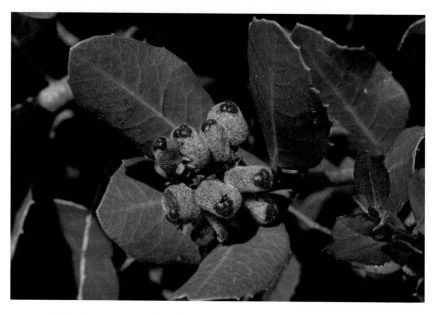

Scientific name – Rhus integrifolia
Common name – lemonade berry, shtoyho'os (pronounced shtoyhokose, Chumash)

Identification – This small tree grows to 24 feet high, but is usually about 10 feet high. The leaves are evergreen, about two inches long and an inch and a half wide. They are elliptic and may have teeth on the edges. The small flowers form in a small panicle and are white or pink. The fruit are round, flat, about a third of an inch long, covered with hairs and are reddish. The flavor of the fruit is sweet and sour, like lemonade (1).

Characteristics – This plant is found in chaparral and favors north facing slopes. It grows to about 2,500 feet in elevation. Lemonade berry has an unfortunate ability to hydridize with sugar bush, making identification sometimes impossible (1).

Distribution – This plant is found in Southern and Baja California (1).

Primary uses – The fruit of lemonade berry is very good tasting and was eaten or mixed with water to make a drink that tastes similar to lemonade. The berries were sucked to alleviate thirst (4).

Secondary uses – It is possible that a leaf tea was made from this plant to treat colds and lung congestion, just as described for R. ovata. Since the two species hybridize, it is sometimes impossible to distinguish the leaves of the two species.

Active compounds – Rhus plants contain many flavones, cardanols and some bichalcones (201-3). Antiviral compounds from Rhus include moronic acid, betulonic acid, robustaflavone and morelloflavone (204). An anticancer compound of current interest is hinokiflavone from Rhus plants (203). Rhus plants contain compounds that are active against bacterial infections such as methyl gallate and gallic acid (205). A possible anti-inflammatory agent, 6-pentadecylsalicylic acid, is found in Rhus plants (206). Rhus plants from Korea and New Zealand are known to contain urushiols that cause allergic reactions and skin rashes (207).

Recommendations – It is highly recommended to use lemonade berries to alleviate thirst. It is probably safe to use a leaf tea to treat colds. Bacterial pneumonia must be diagnosed and treated by a health care provider. Do not treat bacterial pneumonia by yourself.

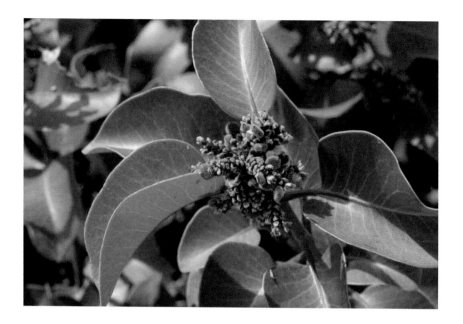

Scientific name – Rhus ovata
Common name – sugar bush

Identification – This small tree grows up to 30 feet high, but is usually about 8 feet high. The leaves are evergreen, ovate and have no teeth. The leaves are usually about two and a half inches long and wide. The small flowers grow in a small panicle and are white or pink. The fruit are round, flat, about a quarter of an inch in diameter, red and covered with hairs (1). The fruit is bitter. The bush and flowers are reported to smell like sugar.

Characteristics – Sugar bush is found in the chaparral below about 4,000 feet in elevation. This plant hydridizes with lemonade berry (1).

Distribution – This plant is found in Southern California, Arizona and Baja California (1).

Primary uses – A tea was made from the leaves for treating colds and other lung infections, and dysmenorrhea. An infusion of the leaves was used to facilitate child birth (4).

Secondary uses – The berries were eaten or mixed with water to make a sweet drink (4).

Active compounds – Refer to Rhus integrifolia.

Recommendations – It is safe to eat the berries of sugar bush. The flavor is not as good as lemonade berries, however. It is probably safe to use a leaf tea from sugar bush, in moderation, to treat colds and dysmenorrhea. For dysmenorrhea, also use a standard anti-inflammatory drug. Bacterial pneumonia must be diagnosed and treated by a health care provider. Child birth is made easier with epidural anesthesia. However, it is probably safe to use a leaf infusion from sugar bush to facilitate child birth.

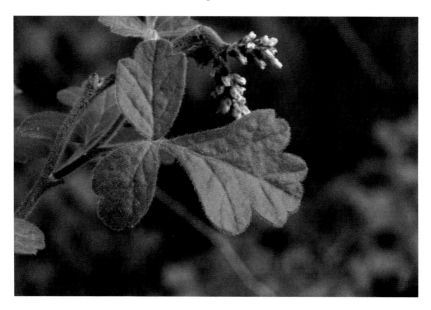

Scientific name – Rhus trilobata
Common name – skunkbrush, basket bush, shu'nay (pronounced shewknay, Chumash)

Identification – This shrub grows up to seven feet tall, but is usually about three feet tall (1). The leaves look very much like small poison oak leaves. There are three leaflets in each leaf.

The only difference with poison oak is that the middle leaflet has only a very short petiole, unlike poison oak where a long petiole is present. Just like poison oak, the leaflets turn brilliant red in the fall and are deciduous. Be very careful in the identification of this plant. The very small flowers form in small panicles and are yellow. The fruit is red-orange, sticky and has a few hairs. It is about one quarter of an inch long and is oblong in shape. The fruit has a mildly sour flavor.

Characteristics – Skunkbrush grows in canyons and north facing slopes below about 6,000 feet in elevation (1).

Distribution – This plant is found in the Western and Central United States as well as Southern Canada and Northern Mexico (1).

Primary uses – A leaf tea was used to treat colds and other lung infections, and stomach ache. The berries were used in the treatment of sores. A leaf decoction was used to wash babies' eyes (4).

Secondary uses – The berries were eaten or dried, ground and made into a soup. Skunkbrush stems were very important in the manufacture of baskets. This plant was used throughout California to make baskets (4).

Active compounds – Refer to Rhus integrifolia.

Recommendations – It is safe to eat the berries. It is probably safe to use a leaf tea from skunkbrush, in moderation, for colds and stomach ache. Bacterial pneumonia must be treated by a health care provider. It is probably safe to mash the berries into a paste and apply it to closed sores. Open sores should be treated with petroleum jelly and antibiotics or steroids. The berry paste may promote bacterial or fungal infections in open sores. Do not wash anyone's eyes with any leaf decoction from any plant. Leaf decoctions contain bacteria, fungi and particles that can be very harmful to eyes. It is safe and very time consuming to make baskets from skunkbrush.

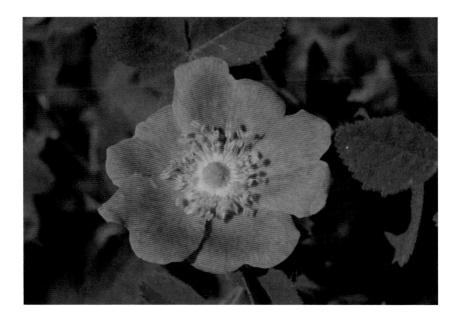

Scientific name - Rosa californica
Common name – California rose, watiqoniqon (pronounced watteekwoanneekwoan, Chumash)

Identification – This shrub is usually about three or four feet tall and can form thickets. The stems are gray-brown and have a few, short, curved prickles. The leaflets are about an inch long, grow in a pinnate formation and are somewhat hairy. The flowers are usually pink with yellow stamens and are about two or three inches wide (1). The flowers can have a very pleasant rose smell and can perfume the woods.

Characteristics – California rose grows throughout the state. It is usually found near streams below about 5,000 feet in elevation (1). The fresh petals taste sweet and perfume the mouth and nose.

Distribution – This plant is found from Oregon to Baja California (1).

Primary uses – A maceration made from mashing the petals of this plant in cold water was useful for colic, teething and constipation in babies. The petals were also dried and crushed to make baby powder. Rose hips were eaten fresh or dried and stored for later use as a food (4, 15).

"California rose was a sweetener. I make a tea to soothe people. It is an internal plant used to lighten someone's load. Drinking the tea relieves anxiety, helps soothe people, so they're not so irritated at the world." Cecilia Garcia (Chumash)

Secondary uses – A tea made from hips or petals was used as an eye wash. A root extract was used for colds. The hips were used to treat pain, fevers, sore throat and kidney problems. The blossoms and powdered roots were used by Cahuilla and Luiseno people as a laxative (4).

Active compounds – Rose petals and leaves contain a number of flavonols, especially derivatives of quercetin and kaempferol (208, 209). Tannins are found in the leaves and petals (209). Catechins are found in the roots (209). Monoterpenes, including the fragrant compounds geraniol, nerol and citronellol, are present in the petals and leaves (209). Monoterpenes are used in the perfume industry. Triterpenes are found in the leaves and roots (209). Sesquiterpenes such as hamanasol and the antifungal carotane, rugosal A are found in the leaves (209). Rose hips are rich in vitamin C (up to 1.7%), beta-carotene, lycopene, tetracyclic triterpene acids, flavonoids and other compounds (3). Oleanolic acid, pomolic acid and their derivatives from rose plants have been shown to be active against HIV (210). Phenoxychromones are found in the leaves. The leaves and seeds contain tocopherols related to vitamin E (209). Sterols, such as sitosterol and campesterol are found in the roots (209).

Recommendations – It is safe, but very labor intensive, to make baby powder from dried rose petals. Discontinue use is a rash results, as this could be due to an allergy to rose petals and pollen. The pleasant maceration made from rose petals may be soothing to babies when given in small sips as a body temperature preparation. It is probably safer to rub rose petal maceration on the gums of a baby for teething than to use the standard, brandy. Tannins in rose petal maceration may be useful as laxatives, in moderation. Dried California rose hips are a pleasant food with a mild, sweet apple flavor. Do not make a tea of rose hips or petals for an eye wash. Particles in the tea may scratch your eye. A tea that has not been boiled enough may contain bacteria and fungi that are dangerous for the eye. It is probably safe to use rose hips or a root tea for the treatment of colds, in moderation. Rose hip tea can probably be safely used for sore throats, pain and fevers. Sesquiterpenes and triterpenes in the plant can be anti-inflammatory and useful against pain. However, high fevers are best treated with drugs known to decrease fevers. Use these drugs only at the recommended doses. Kidney disorders should be treated by a health care provider. Discuss adding rose hip tea to your therapy for kidney disease. Drinking a mild rose petal tea is a safe and soothing way to relax.

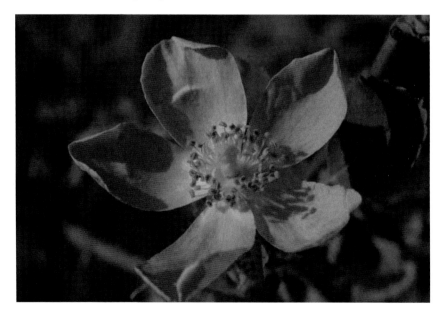

Scientific name - Rosa woodsii
Common name – Interior rose

Identification – This shrub is usually found singly, but can grow in thickets. It usually grows to be about 3 feet tall, but can be much taller in some areas. The stems are usually brown with a few thin, straight prickles. The leaflets are usually about an inch long, grow in a pinnate formation and have no hairs. The flowers are usually red-pink, with yellow stamens and are about four inches wide or less (1). The flowers have a sweet smell of rose that can sometimes create a very pleasant smell.

Characteristics – Interior rose grows in dry areas and can grow in shade or bright sun. It is found in the mountains between about 2,000 and 10,000 feet in elevation (1).

Distribution – This plant is found from British Columbia to Southern California and east to Montana and Nevada (1).

Primary uses – A decoction of the root was used to stop diarrhea by the Paiute and Shoshone. The hips were used as food (79).

Secondary uses – A decoction of the root and bark was used for colds and general debility. It was also used to induce urination. A poultice was made from unspecified parts of the plant for burns and wounds (79).

Active compounds – See R. californica for a discussion of the active compounds in rose plants.

Recommendations – Catechins in the roots can stop diarrhea. To make a decoction, chop up some root, wash it carefully, and add it to a small amount of water. Let it sit for a few hours or overnight. Filter the decoction before drinking. Use this decoction in moderation. Serious diarrhea can be life threatening, especially in children, and should be treated by a health care provider. It is safe to use this decoction, in moderation, for colds and mild debility. Severe debility, such as from a back injury or cancer, should be treated by a health care provider. The hips from interior rose are pleasant food and can be eaten when fresh or dried. Tannins are astringent and can stop bleeding. Interior rose should not be used to make a poultice for burns or wounds, except as a temporary measure. Poultices can be dangerous since they can contain bacteria and fungi from the plant. Always wash wounds with soap and water before applying a clean bandage.

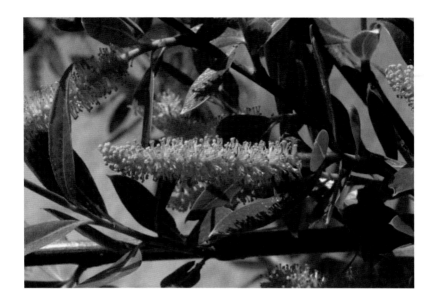

Scientific name – Salix lasiolepis
Common name – arroyo willow, khaw (Chumash)

Identification – This tree reaches as much as 30 feet tall, but is usually about 15 feet tall. The twigs are usually brown. The leaves are more or less lanceolate with wedge shaped bases and tips that are not pointed. The leaves are usually about four inches long and an inch and a quarter wide. They are shiny on the top and covered with powder on the under surface. The inflorescence is called a catkin and appears before the leaves form. The catkin is usually about three inches long (1).

Characteristics – This willow is abundant and is probably the most common willow in California. It is presented here as an example of the many willows found in Southern California. Distinguishing the various species of Salix trees can be difficult. Arroyo willow is usually found in streams (arroyo in Spanish), lake shores, marshes and other wet places. These willows require permanent water. It is found up to 8,000 feet in elevation (1). Willow is a symbol of women for Chumash and other people, because willow is flexible and never breaks.

Primary uses – A tea was made from the bark for fever, colds, sore throat, head aches, pains and malaria. Malaria is discussed under Garrya. The tea was applied to cuts and hemorrhoids. The bark was chewed for tooth aches. Poultices were made from the bark, leaves, twigs and roots to relieve pain, swelling, skin infections and bleeding. Willow seems to have been an important medicinal plant for all California Indians (4).

"Willow can alter the degree of pain and swelling. I mix kelp with willow bark to make a poultice. Willow bark is shredded and left in wet kelp for a couple of days. Then I wrap a swelling with it. The bark can be rolled and burned. It stuns people back into a normal state, especially people who are overwhelmed or whiney." Cecilia Garcia (Chumash)

Secondary uses – An infusion of the leaves was used to induce vomiting. An infusion made from the roots was used to stop diarrhea. The Yuma made a root tea to induce vomiting and cleanse infected blood. The vomiting was so drastic that some did not survive the treatment. Willow poles were used to make frames for houses, acorn granaries, baby carriers, racks, as fire drills and fire hearth sticks. The inner bark of willow was used to make cordage for dance skirts, nets and strings (4). The cordage is derived by burying the bark in gray mud beside a stream for several days until the bark decays leaving the fiber (211).

Active compounds – Willow contains natural salicylates such as salicin, salicortin, tremulacin, populin and others (3). Salicin is converted by intestinal flora to saligenin that is oxidized in the liver to salicylic acid (3). Willow bark can contain up to 10% salicin. Other compounds are present as well including aromatic aldehydes, flavonoids and tannins (3).

Recommendations – It is safe and very useful to chew on willow bark or make a tea from the bark to relieve pains and fevers. Be aware that salicylic acid can irritate the stomach if used in excess. Stomach irritation can be decreased by drinking plenty of water. Excessive use of willow in children can lead to liver failure known as Reye's syndrome. The lukewarm tea can be safely applied to hemorrhoids, aching areas and swollen areas. Poultices from willow can be safely used to treat pain and swelling. Poultices should not be applied to open or bleeding wounds, except as an emergency, temporary measure. Poultices can contain bacteria and fungi. Be sure to wash all wounds with soap and water before applying a clean bandage. Bleeding should be stopped with pressure from the hands, while wearing protective gloves when available. Do not take the time to make a poultice to stop bleeding. The time lost could be dangerous to a bleeding person. It is probably safe to use, in moderation, an infusion made from the roots of willow to stop diarrhea. Do not use willow to induce vomiting. This is very dangerous since inhalation of stomach contents can damage the lungs. It is probably safe to use the smoke from willow bark as aroma therapy, in moderation, to bring people back to a normal state.

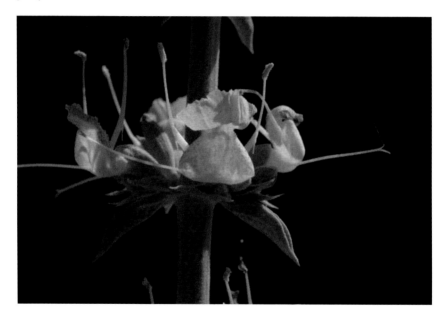

Scientific name – Salvia apiana
Common names – white sage, we'wey (pronounced waykway, Chumash)

Identification – White sage is a shrub that is usually less than 3 feet high, however the flowering stalks can grow to 6 feet high. The leaves are oblong or lanceolate and are 2 to 3 inches long. The mature leaves have a characteristic silver green color. The white flowers are about one half inch long and have long stamens and styles that emerge from the flowers (1).

Characteristics – White sage is a perennial and is found in sunny, chapparal areas in the foothills below about 4,000 feet. The leaves have a pungent sage smell and a soothing, sage flavor. The flowers appear from April to June (1).

Distribution – This plant is found in Southern and Baja California (1).

Primary uses – The leaves of this plant had many uses including for sore throat and, especially among the Luiseno and Cahuilla, as shampoo (4). The use of shampoo is critical in the control of head lice, a major problem among Mission Indians. Mission Indians were not allowed to bathe, which created skin and hair problems for those Indians who were used to bathing everyday (15). The Chumash custom was to bathe every morning before the sun rose. A drink was made by putting a leaf in cold water to promote strengthening, and cure colds and flus. This drink was used every day. White sage leaves were used as a deodorant to remove human smells during deer hunting, either by rubbing the leaves on the skin or by chewing the leaves. After a night of prayer and fasting in the sweat lodge, the men would wash and dress in deer skins with the deer heads stuffed full of tule. Camouflaged and deodorized, they went to hunt. White sage leaves were also eaten to repair the soul.

"It is our everyday plant. It is a spirit plant. If you don't have it, everything is going to bother you. You drink it by putting a leaf in cool water everyday. You are going to be calm enough to be rational. It will enhance any medicine you take and protect you from the toxicity of medicines. It tickles your spirit, your conscience, and helps you keep your integrity. If you drink it everyday, you won't get as many colds. Some people have very harsh communication skills. If they smoke white sage, they're just a little gentler. If drug addicts smoke it, it helps give them direction. They're not aggressive. It cures their addictions one hundred percent. If you are very sick, drink sage tea. The water has to start at room temperature. Heat it until it just starts to boil. It must be tended so it doesn't boil, or it will loose its effect."

Cecilia Garcia (Chumash)

Secondary uses – The uses of white sage were numerous including to treat sore throat, stomach ache, tooth ache, asthma, to promote menstruation and to cleanse wounds. The root was used to promote healing after child birth. The seeds and young stems were eaten as food. The leaves were sometimes smoked, perhaps to induce sacred dreams, hallucinations. The leaves were burned or smudged to invite good spirits and to drive away evil spirits (4).

"When you burn white sage you have to pray. You're supposed to be healing someone. You're supposed to be at attention, because white sage is our protection. If you're not praying, someone is not being protected." Cecilia Garcia (Chumash)

Active compounds – Plants of the genus Salvia contain cineole (eucalyptol) that is soothing to the throat (3). There are several other monoterpenoids in this plant that, like cineole, are also pain relievers. A large number of active diterpenoids are found in Salvia (212). Some Salvia diterpenoids are active against diarrhea or are antibiotics (213). At least one diterpene, salvinorin A, is a potent hallucinogen, that can be smoked (214). Please read the section on Sacred not Psychedelic later in this book. The anti-allergic activities of some Salvias are due to diterpenoids. Some Salvia diterpenoids are active against tuberculosis (215). Another Salvia compound, miltirone, may act like vallium to relieve anxiety (216). Salvia also contains thujone (3) that is hallucinogenic, addictive and induces convulsions as discussed under Artemesia douglasiana.

Recommendation – White sage can be used safely to relieve sore throat simply by sucking on a fresh leaf for a few minutes. A shampoo can be made by rubbing fresh leaves between the palms with water. This may be where the idea for commercially available, herbal shampoo was derived. Using white sage as a deodorant is safe and effective. It is probably safe to use white sage decoction in moderation during colds and flus, or to prevent these conditions. It is also probably safe to use white sage in moderation for stomach ache, tooth ache and to promote healing and menstruation. Asthma is a serious condition that should be treated with drugs known to be effective. It may be safe to use white sage for asthma, in combination with standard drugs for asthma. Inform your health care provider before adding white sage to your asthma therapy. The presence of thujone in white sage makes the plant potentially dangerous for long term use or smoking. There are reports of California Indians smoking white sage with no deleterious effects or sacred dreams, hallucinations. It may be necessary to smoke a large amount of white sage in order to induce a hallucination. Increasing the amount smoked increases the likelihood of convusions and potential death from thujone. However, the potential ability of white sage to stop addictions may be a real benefit to our society. Smudging white sage is safe, provided that inhalation of large amounts of smoke is avoided. To smudge white sage, say a prayer, pick a small branch, let it dry for a few days, then smudge it slowly while praying. Our society could benefit from a plant that helps repair the soul, make us gentler and more communicative. Perhaps prayer, fasting and drinking white sage preparations, in moderation, could help our spirits.

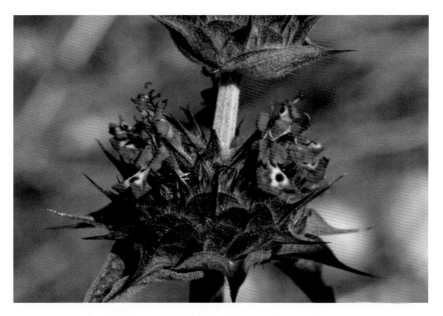

Scientific name – Salvia columbariae
Common names – Chia, 'ilepesh (pronounced gheelaypaysh,

Chumash)

Identification – Chia is a small plant that grows from one to one and a half feet tall. The leaves grow mostly at the base in a ragged, pinnate formation and are about 3 to 6 inches long. The very small, purple flowers grow in large clusters on the stalk and appear from March to June. When the flowers wither, the remaining clusters are full of very small, black seeds. The plant may have a mild sage smell and flavor.

Characteristics – Chia is an annual plant and grows in the Spring, blooming in April. It is found in chaparral areas below about 4,000 feet (1). Chia was planted and carefully cultivated by California Indians wherever they lived. After the harvest, the area was burned to increase the crop the next year (15).

Distribution – This plant is found in California, Nevada, Utah and Arizona (1).

Primary uses – Chia was a food plant. The seeds were eaten or mixed with water and drunk (4). According to Chumash legends, the root, leaves or stalk was used to revive people who were almost dead (72). It is not known which sick people were revived with chia, perhaps heart attack or stroke victims.

Secondary uses – Messengers, ksen in Chumash, ate chia seeds to help maintain their endurance on long runs (15, 217). The ksen may have run as much as 30 or 40 miles in a day to deliver messages. The seeds of chia and other sages were used to clean the eye. A seed was placed under the eye lid and allowed to stay in place for several hours or overnight (4,15). This is a dangerous practice that can lead to bacterial infection of the eye and should never be done.

Active compounds – Chia seeds are a source of protein (20%), oil (34%) and other nutrients (4). The seeds may be covered with mucoproteins or polysaccharides that make the seeds very gelatinous when combined with water. The sugars released during digestion of mucoproteins or polysaccharides would be beneficial to endurance runners, as would be the protein. Chia root has recently been found to contain diterpenoids called tanshinones

(218) that increase blood flow. This may be beneficial to stroke, angina and heart attack victims. Compounds that inhibit blood clotting, such as salvianolic acid A, are present in some Salvia plants and could be beneficial in stroke (219). Thujone is probably present in chia and can cause hallucinations and seizures.

Recommendations – Salvia multiorrhiza, dan shen (Chinese), has revolutionized the treatment of heart attack and stroke in China. Dan shen apparently greatly increases the survival of heart attack and stroke, due to the tanshinones present in the plant. The utility of chia in heart attack, angina and stroke is unknown at this time. People suffering from heart attack or stroke should be taken immediately to an emergency room. It is safe and nutritious to use chia seeds for food. The seeds can be bought in many grocery stores.

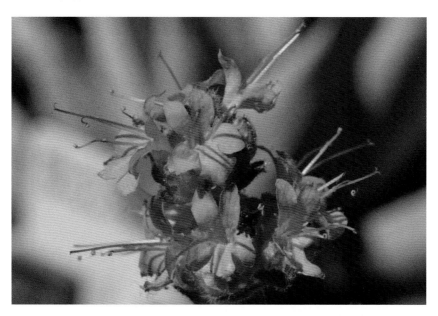

Scientific name – Salvia dorii
Common name – gray ball sage

Identification – It is usually found as a small shrub up to two and a half feet high. The stem and leaves are covered with white scales. The leaves are usually spoon shaped and about an inch and a half long. The tubular flowers grow in clusters and are usually blue. Large, purple bracts grow among the flower clusters (1).

Characteristics – Gray ball sage is a perennial and is found in dry places up to 7,000 feet in elevation (1). Although found in the desert, this is not a strictly desert plant. The leaves have a mild sage smell and taste. This is the plant sometimes inappropriately called purple sage.

Distribution – This plant is found throughout the Great Basin in Washington, Oregon, Idaho, Utah, Nevada, California and Arizona (1).

Primary uses – The leaves and stems of this sage was eaten by the Kawaiisu to cure stomach aches or drunk as a decoction to cure colds. The leaves were also smoked with tobacco to cure colds (4).

Secondary uses – The dried leaves were smoked to clear nasal congestion. The Paiute used a leaf decoction against venereal diseases. The Kawaiisu burned gray ball sage leaves to drive away evil spirits (4).

Active compounds – Some Salvia species contain cineole and camphor that can soothe the stomach (3). Diterpenoids such as secoisopimarane are present in sages and can relax gut smooth muscle (220). This activity would help relieve aches in the guts. Salvias contain norditerpenoids and diterpene quinones that are active against tuberculosis and bacteria (215, 221). Their activities against viruses and venereal diseases are unknown. There are tanshinones in Salvias that affect the immune system (222). This may be beneficial against colds and venereal diseases.

Recommendations – Salvia dorii can probably be used safely against colds and stomach aches, in moderation. Venereal diseases should be treated with prescription drugs. Discuss with your health care provider adding Salvia dorii to standard therapy for venereal diseases. These diseases probably occurred in California before the Europeans arrived, but greatly increased when the Indians were forced to live in Missions. It is not recommended to smoke gray ball sage, especially in combination with tobacco. Smoking can lead to lung damage and emphysema. It is safe to carefully smudge gray ball sage leaves to drive away evil spirits, especially if it works.

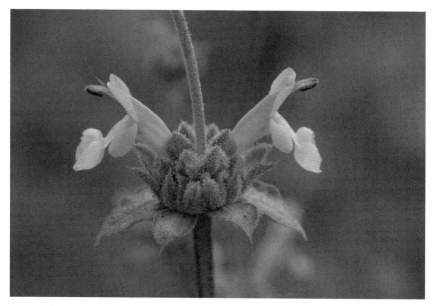

Scientific name – Salvia mellifera
Common name – Black sage

Identification – Black sage is a shrub between 3 and 6 feet high. The rough, elliptical leaves are usually an inch or an inch and a half long. The blue flowers grow in clusters on the stem. The flowers are about half an inch long (1). The entire plant has a pungent sage smell and taste.

Characteristics – The plant is a perennial and grows in chaparral areas up to about 3,000 feet in elevation (1). It can be very common in some areas. Flowers bloom from April to July.

Distribution – This plant is found in California and Baja California (1).

Primary uses – Black sage leaves were used to relieve pain,

perhaps due to anti-inflammatory agents present in the plant. A decoction of the plant was used as a bath for arthritic limbs. Either black sage or purple sage (Salvia leucophylla) leaves were soaked in water to make a decoction. The patient was instructed to place the arthritic hand or foot on a deer antler or bone in a bath of the sage decoction. The patient carefully moved the hand or foot on the antler for a massage while soaking for fifteen minutes or so.

"I put my feet on top of the deer antler to loosen the feet, that connect everything in the body. I really like the way it feels. Sometimes I get juniper or cedar and mix them with black sage. I throw it in a blender until it's like dust. I put that in my shoes to relieve pain." Cecilia Garcia (Chumash)

"Black sage (Kasili, Tongva) was often combined with white sage for blessing ceremonies." Julia Bogany (Tongva)

Secondary uses – Black sage was one of the most widely used spices for flavoring foods. Colic, coughs, sore throats and ear aches were treated with the plant (4).

Active compounds – Some Salvia plants contain anti-inflammatory compounds such as aethiopinone and ursolic acid (223, 224). Thujone is also present in this plant and can be hallucinogenic, addictive and cause seizures.

Recommendation – There is a constant need for new, less irritating anti-inflammatory agents. Black sage may provide moderate pain relief. It is safe to use as a spice, for colic in babies, for coughs, for sore throats and for pain relief, in moderation. Ear infections should be treated with antibiotic drugs. Black sage should not be smoked or extracted with alcohol, since smoking damages the lungs and alcoholic extracts would contain thujone.

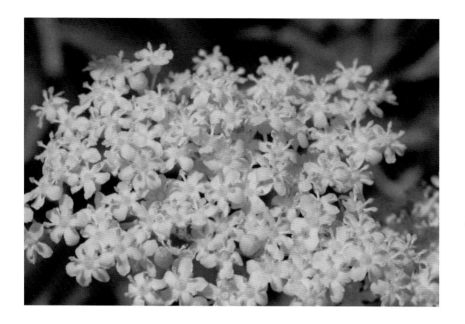

Scientific name – Sambucus mexicana
Common names – Elderberry, tree of music

Identification – Elderberry grows as a shrub or tree up to 25 feet tall. There are many elliptical leaflets, 2 – 3 inches long, in a pinnate arrangement. In the Spring, the small, white flowers grow in large panicles (1). The fruit are small, spherical berries about one quarter inch or less in diameter. They form in the Spring and Summer and can be white or purple when ripe. The fruit is sweet when it is dried.

Characteristics – Elderberry is a perennial and is common along streams, in the forest and in chaparral (1). Deer frequently find shelter under the drooping limbs. Elderberry may have been planted by California Indians to mark places where springs or underground water could be found.

Distribution – This plant grows throughout the west from British Columbia to Southern California, Utah and New Mexico (1).

Primary uses – A tea made from elderberry flowers was used by most California Indians to cure colds and flus. It was used against fevers as well. The inner bark was used as an emetic. The fresh berries, but not the dried berries, can cause nausea in some people (4). The branches were used to make clapper sticks (217). These are split sticks, with a sound chamber at one end, that make a sharp sound when struck against the open palm. Clapper sticks were used instead of drums by many California Indians. Flutes were sometimes made from elderberry sticks.

"Elderberry is the music tree, our heartbeat. It helps restore the normal flow. I use the leaves, berries, flowers and bark to make a mild tea that gets the normal flow going in the body." Cecilia Garcia (Chumash)

Secondary uses – The berries were dried and used as food. They have a very sweet and pleasant taste, like currants. The berries were also used as a laxative and to make wine. Blossom tea was used to relieve premenstrual syndrome and dysmenorrhea. A dark purple dye was made from the twigs and fruit to dye basketry. The small branches were sometimes used to make arrow shafts. The flowers were used to make shampoo by rubbing the flowers between the palms with a little water. Shampoos were very important to California Indians in the control of lice (4).

Active compounds – Elderberry is a good source of vitamin C (3). Other active constituents include rutin, ebulin, lectins, triterpenoids such as lupeol, sterols such as beta-sitosterol, flavonoids such as the anthocyanin cyanidin-3-sambubuioside, glycosides, tannins and aromas such as cis-rose oxide (3). The bark, roots and leaves contain a cyanogenic glycoside that can cause nausea, vomiting and diarrhea (3). This glycoside is potentially dangerous if used in large amounts. Sambucol, a standardized Sambucus nigra extract, is available in Europe and has been shown in clinical trials to decrease the duration of the flu by 3 to 4 days (225). Sambucol appears to increase the immune response against viral infections, even HIV (226). An aqueous extract of Sambucus has insulin-like activity, stimulates insulin release and may be useful against diabetes (227). This extract also has diuretic properties (228). An extract of Sambucus ebulus is active against pain and inflammation (229). An extract of Sambucus sieboldiana, which contains vanillic acid, inhibits bone resoption and may be useful against osteoporosis (230).

Recommendation – The dried berries are sweet and should be eaten. The blossom tea is widely recognized by California Indians as effective against colds and flus. It should be used. To make the tea, use one teaspoon of dried or fresh elderberry blossoms in one and a half cups of boiling water. Let it steep for about 5 minutes. Add sugar and drink. The flavor is not particularly pleasant, but is tolerable. The tea should be used once a day for the first 3 to 5 days of a cold or flu. Recent clinical trials of a product from Sambucus nigra, from South America, have shown that it decreases the duration of colds and flus. The dried berries can be safely used as a laxative. Elderberry wine is very pleasant and should be drunk in moderation. The blossom tea can be safely used, in moderation, for premenstrual syndrome and dysmenorrhea. Standard anti-inflammatory drugs should also be used for dysmenorrhea. It is safe to use elderberry blossom shampoo. It is not recommended to use elderberry to regulate heart beat. This should be done with drugs known to be effective.

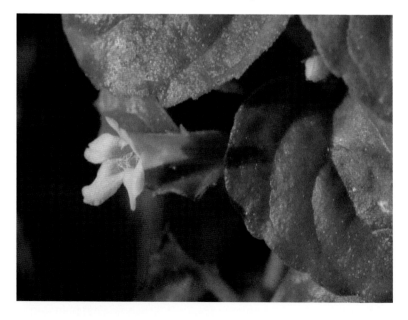

Scientific name – Satureja douglasii
Common names – Yerba Buena (Spanish).

Identification – This is a small, low growing vine that tends to grow in mats. The stems are usually green, but can be brown and woody. The leaves are ovate and about three quarters of an inch long. The margins have small teeth. The flowers are small, white tubes about a quarter of an inch long (1). The leaves smell of mint and have a pleasant, sweet taste.

Characteristics – Yerba Buena is a very nonspecific name that is applied to any plant that smells or tastes like mint. Satureja douglasii used to be common and was found in shady places in chaparral and forests below 2,500 feet in elevation (1). It is usually found on steep slopes growing underneath the poison oak. The original name of San Francisco is Yerba Buena. However, grazing, development and introduced plants have greatly diminished the places this plant can be found. It is now a rare plant in Southern California and can no longer be found on Yerba Buena road in the Santa Monica Mountains.

Distribution – This plant is found from British Columbia and Idaho to Southern California (1).

Primary uses – Satureja douglasii was used to treat parasitic worm infections (15). These infections were apparently mostly from tapeworms (cestodes). The Chumash and most other Indians ate raw fish that were probably the source of the tapeworms. Of course, ocean fish are usually not infested with tapeworms. Fresh water fish are more commonly infested with tapeworms. Eating bear meat and marine mammal meat can cause trichinosis from nematode (round worm) infestation of the meat. The Chumash and other sea coast people ate whale, sea lion and seal meat. Eating bear meat was rare in California, since the primary bear was the grizzly bear. But on those occasions when a grizzly bear was killed, bear meat was eaten. The usual rule was that the bear won the fight, not the Indian. Spanish and American hunters caused the extinction of the bear. Grizzly bears have been extinct in California since 1922 and can only be seen on the state flag.

Secondary uses – A tea made from the leaves of Satureja douglasii was used to treat stomach ache, gas, colic in babies, for colds, fevers, tooth ache, insomnia, urinary tract problems, to promote menstruation and for menstrual cramps (4, 15). The leaves were also used as a deodorant before hunting, in much the same way white sage was used (4).

Active compounds – Satureja species contain many active flavonoids that are antimicrobial against bacteria and fungi (231, 232). Extracts of Satureja species have been shown to kill HIV and other viruses (233). The essential oils of some Satureja species relax smooth muscles (antispasmodic) and can help against diarrhea (234). Eriodictyol, naringenin and luteolin are flavonoids found in Satureja species that are vasodilators and could decrease blood pressure (235).

Recommendations – It is safe and very pleasant to drink, in moderation, a mild tea made from Satureja douglasii. The tea is mildly sweet and may have a strong mint smell. Please grow this plant in your garden and refrain from collecting it in the wild. The tea could be soothing in stomach ache, gas, colic, colds, fever, tooth ache, insomnia, and menstrual cramps. Drinking fluids is in general helpful for urinary tract problems. It is not safe to promote menstruation in a pregnant woman. However, Satureja douglasii tea should be soothing for women just starting their periods. Tapeworm and round worm infections are serious conditions that should be treated by a health care provider. Talk to your health care provider about adding Satureja douglasii to your therapy for these infections. Maybe someday, drugs made from Satureja douglasii will be available for these infections. It is safe to use this plant as a deodorant, if you want to smell like mint.

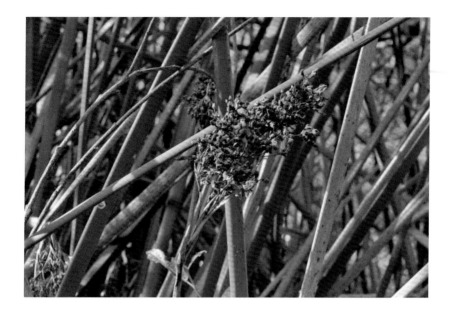

Scientific name - Scirpus acutus occidentalis
Common name – Tule (pronounced tulee)

Identification – This plant is usually about six feet tall and grows from long rhizomes. The stems are cylindric and about half an inch in diameter. The leaves are basal, small and not usually seen. The inflorescence is a panicle at the top of the stem that is about three inches long and made up of many brown spikeletts (1).

Characteristics – This common plant is found almost anywhere permanent ponds or lakes occur. It is found up to 7,500 feet in elevation. It grows in dense communities along the edges of ponds and lakes (1).

Distribution – This plant grows throughout North America (1).

Primary use – Tule was used to make thatched houses called tules, casts, baby carriers, canoes called balsas, diapers, skirts, mats and water bottles. The Chumash made elevated sleeping mats, beds, from tule (217). Casts were made by wrapping tule around and along the broken bone and applying glue made from asphaltum, pine sap and soap root lily (15). The cast dried hard and black. The patient was sometimes anesthetized with momoy or Solanum douglasii when the bone was set.

Active compounds – This plant was used structurally, not as a medicine.

Recommendations – It is safe to use tule. However, no one knows how to make tule casts anymore, since the recipe for the glue is no longer known. This may have been similar to the glue used to make canoes. It is easier to go to the emergency room to have a broken bone treated.

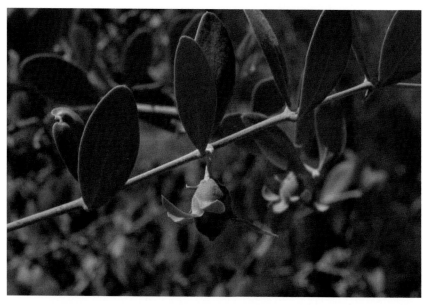

Scientific name – Simmondsia chinensis
Common name – Jojoba (Spanish), goat nut, pig nut

Identification – This bush grows to about five feet tall and has spreading branches. The leaves are dull green, opposite, ovate and have very short petioles. The flowers are small and have five green sepals. The fruit is a green nut about a third of an inch wide (1).

Characteristics – Jojoba is found in arid areas of the desert below about 4,500 feet in elevation (1). The seeds contain liquid wax.

Distribution – This plant is found in Southern California, Arizona and Northern Mexico (1).

Primary uses – The nuts were eaten fresh or boiled (4, 12, 67). When roasted, they apparently have a flavor like hazelnuts (4).

Secondary uses – Kumeyaay and other desert people derived liquid wax from the nuts that was rubbed on the hair and skin as a shampoo and lotion (12, 67). A jojoba preparation was drunk by women near the time of birth to provide an easier delivery (12).

Active compounds – Jojoba contains wax that is used commercially in the cosmetics industry (236). Jojoba is cultivated in several countries for wax production. The nuts contain proteins and cyanomethylene glycosides called simmondsins (237). Simmondsins fed to animals cause loss of appetite and anemia (238).

Recommendations – Many cosmetics contain jojoba wax. It is safe to use these cosmetics, in moderation. It is safe to use the liquid wax as a skin lotion. It is not recommended to eat the fresh nuts in large amounts, since they may cause anemia. It is not known if roasting or boiling destroys the simmondsins in the nuts. Therefore, it is not recommended to eat the roasted or boiled nuts in large amounts. It is not recommended to drink a jojoba preparation near the time of delivery since anemia may result.

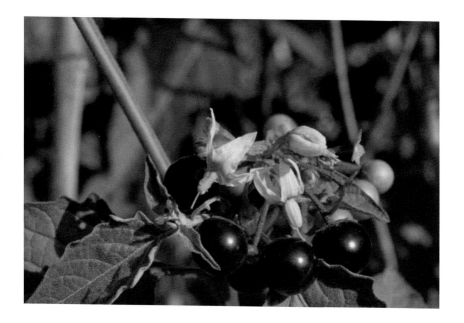

Scientific name – Solanum douglasii
Common name – nightshade

Identification – Nightshade is a small shrub with ovate leaves. The leaves are about three inches long. The flowers grow in an umbel and have white petals with green and yellow centers. The flowers have five fused petals that grow as an open bowl about three quarters of an inch wide. The fruit is a shiny, dark purple fruit about a third of an inch in diameter (1).

Characteristics – This is a fairly common plant in the chaparral and forests below about 3,000 feet in elevation (1). It blooms in July and August.

Distribution – This plant is found in Southern California and Northern Mexico (1).

Primary uses – This plant and Solanum xanti may have been used similarly. S. xanti has purple flowers, with yellow centers and green fruit. The plant was used to induce a stupor under which the patient was insensitive to painful procedures.

"The berries were fermented to make a heavy, syrupy wine. If a broken bone had to be moved back in place, that berry stuff would desensitize the person." Cecilia Garcia (Chumash)

Active compounds – Solanum plants contain many steroidal alkaloids such as solanine and chaconine (239). Solanine was used medicinally in the past in asthma, bronchitis and epilepsy. Some steroids, perhaps including nightshade steroids, have anesthetic activity. Solanum steroidal alkaloids induce nausea, diarrhea, gut lesions and have anticholinergic activity (240). This activity can result in hallucinations, stupor, dilated pupils, fever and other symptoms. However, the ripe berries may be safer to eat than the unripe berries. Apparently, the unripe berries can have higher concentrations of solanine than the ripe berries. The Chumash and other Indians have been reported to eat the ripe berries as food (4, 61). Eating the berries can cause fetal malformation in animals (239). This plant should not be confused with Atropa belladonna, deadly nightshade, that has killed many people.

Recommendations – It is not safe to use nightshade berries to induce a stupor. This can easily kill the person. Anesthesia should only be induced by an Anesthesiologist who is trained in how to monitor and treat patients in a stupor. The ripe berries have a pleasant, sweet flavor, but must be eaten with caution. Eat only one berry and wait twenty minutes before eating another berry. If nausea occurs, stop eating the berries. Women who may be pregnant should not eat the berries.

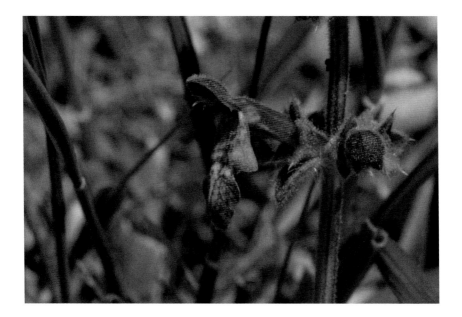

Scientific name –Stachys bullata
Common name – hedge nettle

Identification – This plant is usually about a foot tall and grows from a single stem. The leaves are ovate, covered with hair and about two and a half inches long. The flowers grow in spikes, are pink, and are made of a tube with a prominent lower lip. The tube is about a quarter of an inch long (1).

Characteristics – This plant is usually found growing in full shade in canyons near the coast. It is common in the Santa Monica Mountains below about 1,500 feet in elevation (1). It blooms in April and May.

Distribution – This plant occurs near the coast from Central to Southern California (1). However, there are other Stachys species that occur throughout the west.

Primary uses – A leaf decoction was used externally as a disinfectant, on skin irritations and sores. It was used internally for stomach aches, coughs and sore throats (4).

Secondary uses – The leaves were warmed and placed on the ear for ear ache. The leaves were bundled to make stoppers for water bottles (4).

Active compounds – Stachys species are used as anti-inflammatory and antibacterial medicines in Europe, China and Africa. The genus has been extensively studied and contains flavonoids, saponins, phenylpropanoids, iridoids, diterpenes, triterpenes, and many other compounds (241-4). Some of the compounds are anti-inflammatory agents (245). Other compounds are active against bacteria (246). However, sheep grazing on Stachys plants in New Zealand and Australia develop peripheral neuropathy, myopathy and may die (247).

Recommendations – It is probably safe to use hedge nettle preparations externally. Discontinue use if a rash forms. It is probably safe to place a warm leaf on the ear to treat ear ache. It is not recommended to use hedge nettle internally or as a stopper for water bottles, due to possible toxicity.

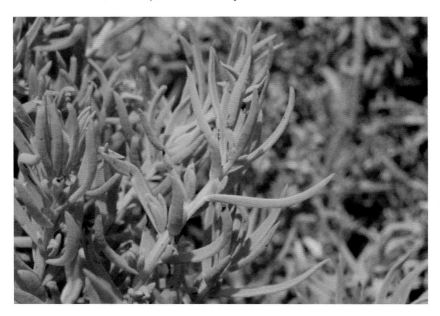

Scientific name – Suaeda esteroa

Common name – Estuary sea blite

Identification – This small shrub grows to about two feet tall. The leaves are fleshy, sessile, linear and about three quarters of an inch long. The upper leaves are green, fleshy and taste like sea water. The lower leaves are tan and withered. The very small flowers grow along the stem in clusters, between the leaves. The black, biconvex seeds are about one eighth of an inch wide (1).

Characteristics – This plant is becoming rare due to habitat destruction. It used to grow along estuaries and salt mashes on the coast (1). This prime land is being developed at the expense of this plant. All of the Suaeda species, even the desert species, were used for their seeds.

Distribution – This plant is found in Southern California and Northern Mexico (1). However, other Suaeda species are found throughout the west.

Primary uses – Estuary sea blite seeds were parched by putting them in a basket with hot rocks. The basket had to be kept in constant motion to avoid charring the basket. The seeds were called pinole and were eaten as is or pounded and formed into cakes. Seeds of other plants, such as Atriplex, were sometimes added to this important food (4).

Secondary uses – Estuary sea blite was burned to produce ashes that were used to make soap (4). Cleanliness was very important to the Chumash people who bathed every day before the sun came up.

Active compounds – Suaeda species contain triterpenoids, sterols and unusual pigments such as citry-celosianin (248, 249). Suaeda extracts have been shown to lower blood glucose and cholesterol levels in laboratory rats (250, 251).

Recommendations – It is safe to eat the seeds of Suaeda plants, as the Indians have done for centuries. It is also safe to use soap made from the plant. It can be purchased from some nurseries to grow at home.

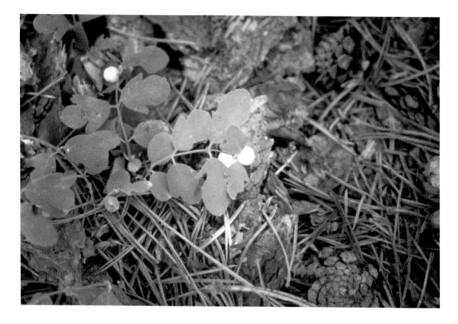

Scientific name – Symphoricarpos mollis
Common name – creeping snowberry, trip vine

Identification – This vine has opposite leaves that are elliptical and about an inch long. The flowers form in small racemes of two to eight flowers that hang down from the stem. The flowers are pink, bell shaped and about a quarter of an inch long. The berries are round, white and about a third of an inch in diameter (1).

Characteristics – Creeping snowberry is found especially in shady, wooded canyons up to 9,000 feet in elevation (1). It is usually found growing on other plants. But can also be found creeping along the ground.

Distribution – This plant is found throughout the west from British Columbia to California and east to Idaho and New Mexico (1).

Primary uses – Infusions of snowberry were used to treat sores and other skin lesions (4).

Secondary uses – Root infusions were used to treat colds and stomach aches (4).

Active compounds – Symphoricarpos species contain many compounds such as beta-sitosterol, oleanolic acid and chelidonine (252, 253). Beta-sitosterol can be useful against skin problems. Oleanolic acid can protect against stomach ulcers, liver damage and has antiviral activity against HIV in laboratory tests (254-6). It has not been tested in patients. Chelidonine inhibits dopaminergic activity in the brain and may be responsible for the vomiting and delirium reported from eating snowberries from Symphoricarpos albus (257, 258).

Recommendations – It is probably safe to use creeping snowberry infusions on sores and other skin lesions. Discontinue use if a rash forms. It is not recommended to use creeping snowberry preparations internally since they may cause vomiting and delirium. Children have died from eating snowberries.

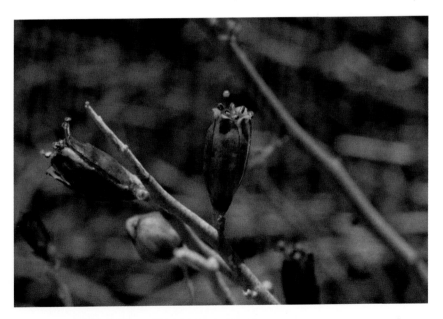

Scientific name – Thamnosma montana
Common name – Turpentine broom

Identification – This broom like plant grows to about two feet tall. The stems are yellowish green and covered with blister like glands. The leaves are usually not seen because they are very small and ephemeral. The flowers are purple tubes about half an inch long. The fruit is a leathery capsule that is deeply divided in two and about half an inch wide (1).

Characteristics – Turpentine broom grows on dry slopes in the desert, especially the desert mountains, below 2,000 feet in elevation (1). The fruit is oily and has an acrid, grapefruit smell. It is very bitter tasting.

Distribution – This plant is found in California, Arizona, Nevada, New Mexico and Mexico (1).

Primary uses – The oil from the fruit was rubbed on the skin to promote healing. A tea made from the stems was used as a tonic, against colds and chest pain (4).

Secondary uses – The roots were used against snake bites and as snake repellants. The roots were claimed to be hallucinogenic. Shamans drank a preparation made from the plant and became temporarily crazy and clairvoyant. However, the preparation could also be fatal (4).

Active compounds – Turpentine broom contains acridone alkaloids, psoralens, coumarins and other compounds (259, 260). The psoralens can cause phototoxicity (261), which is a rash that forms when the skin is exposed to the sun after touching or eating the plant.

Recommendations – It is not recommended to use this plant since it can cause phototoxicity. There are safer plants and drugs to use for skin healing, colds and chest pain. Poisonous snake bites should be treated with antivenom in the emergency room. It is not recommended to carry a piece of the root as a snake repellant since it can cause phototoxicity. It is not recommended to use this plant as a hallucinogen since it can be fatal. However, this practice is protected by religious freedom laws.

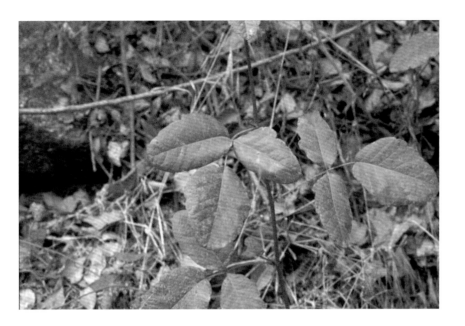

Scientific name – Toxicodendron diversilobum
Common name – poison oak

Identification – This plant grows as a shrub up to 12 feet high or
vine up to 75 feet long. The leaves are made of three leaflets
about two and a half inches long. The margins are usually wavy.
The center leaflet has a petiole about a half inch long. The leaves
turn red in the fall. The very small yellow, green flowers grow as
a droopy raceme. The fruit is white and about a quarter inch in
diameter (1).

Characteristics – This is an abundant plant in the chaparral and
forests. It likes shady, moist areas below about 5,000 feet in
elevation (1).

Distribution – This plant is found from British Columbia to Baja
California (1).

Primary uses – Poison oak was used for many skin problems
including warts, ring worm, and rattlesnake bites (4, 15).

"I have eaten the leaves and never get a rash. Eating the leaves helps prevent skin infections and venereal disease sores. Chumash didn't have the skin infections until the Spanish and venereal diseases and all that. Eat the leaves to prevent infections." Cecilia Garcia (Chumash)

Secondary uses – "Sometimes the minds of Vietnam Veterans were in a shock. A tea of the leaves was used to make them vomit and wake them up. Then they were alive again." Cecilia Garcia (Chumash)

Active compounds – Urushiols are present in poison oak that cause contact dermatitis, rashes. The rash usually lasts for a week or so. Rashes can also form on the mouth when eating poison oak. Urushiols can cause the esophagus to swell and the airways to swell. When the airways swell, breathing can be impossible. This is a common way that fire fighters die, following inhalation of poison oak smoke.

Recommendations – Some people cannot become desensitized to poison oak. They develop the rash every time they contact poison oak. Other people quickly become desensitized and do not develop a rash on the second or third contact of the year with poison oak. These people can even eat the berries and report that they taste good. Other people should never eat the berries or drink a poison oak leaf tea because of the danger of esophageal or airway swelling. It is safe to use poison oak for warts and other skin problems only if you know you will not develop a rash. Ring worm, rattlesnake bite, venereal diseases and skin infections should be treated by a health care provider. It is not safe to use anything to induce vomiting, since inhalation of stomach contents can damage the lungs.

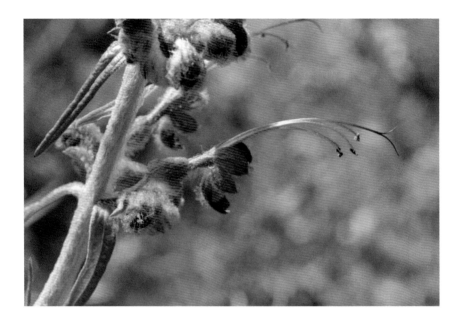

Scientific name – Trichostema lanatum
Common name – Woolly bluecurls, romero (Spanish), 'akhiye'p
(pronounced gokheyaikp, Chumash)

Identification – This plant grows as a shrub, less than four and a
half feet tall. The leaves are linear with the edges rolled under
and very short petioles. The upper surface of the leaves is green.
The under side of the leaves is gray with small hairs. The showy
flowers grow out of woolly blue hairs. The purple flowers are inch
long tubes with long, arched stamens that exert out of the flower
(1).

Characteristics - The leaves have a pungent smell somewhat like
turpentine and sage. The flowers have been described to smell
like hops. The plant grows in chaparral below about 2,400 feet
(1).

Distribution – This plant is found in Southern and Baja California
(1).

Primary uses – Woolly bluecurl flowers were considered a general remedy for many diseases. A tea made from the flowers and leaves was used for stomach aches (4). The tea was considered to be effective against nervous problems, suggesting that it may relieve anxiety, like benzodiazepine drugs. It was also used to darken and strengthen the hair (16).

Secondary uses – The Kumeyaay used this plant to treat colds. The Chumash used it as a douche, especially after child birth. The plant may be a mild fish poison or narcotic, which makes fish easier to catch perhaps by stupefying them (4). The leaves have been routinely used as a spice in foods, with a flavor like rosemary (16).

Active compounds – Plants of the genus Trichostema have a number of aromatic and flavorful compounds, including sabinene, thujene, pinene, myrcene, phellandrene, terpinene, caryophyllene, octenol and other compounds (262). These compounds all contribute to the smell and taste of the plant. The compounds in the plant that are effective against nervous conditions are not reported.

Recommendations – It is safe to use woolly bluecurls as a spice, in shampoos to treat the hair, and as a douche. It is probably safe to use in moderation as a tea to treat stomach aches and colds. Fish poisoning is illegal in most areas. Serious nervous conditions should be treated by a health care provider. Always inform your health care provider whenever you want to add any natural product to your drug therapy.

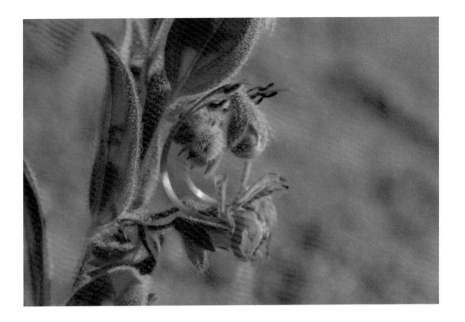

Scientific name – Trichostema lanceolatum
Common name – Vinegar weed

Identification – This small plant grows to less than 3 feet tall and is covered with hairs. The leaves have very short petioles, are lanceolate and about 2 inches long. The blue flowers are tubes, almost an inch long, with exerted stamens that strongly arch back toward the stem (1).

Characteristics - The plant has a very strong smell of vinegar and sage. It is found in dry, grassy areas below about 3,000 feet (1).

Distribution – This plant is found from Oregon to Baja California (1).

Primary uses – The Costanoans, Tubatulabal and Kawaiisu used this plant to treat colds and reduce fevers. It was also used to treat malaria. See Garrya for a discussion of malaria. It was used as a pain reliever especially in tooth ache, stomach ache and head ache (4).

Secondary uses – Vinegar weed was used for uterine problems, nose bleeds, as an insecticide and disinfectant (4).

Active compounds – The active compounds in Trichostema plants include sabinene, thujene, pinene, myrcene, phellandrene, terpinene, caryophyllene, octenol and other compounds (262). The pain relieving, fever reducing and coagulant compounds in this plant are not reported.

Recommendations – This plant can be safely used in moderation to treat colds and minor fevers, simply by chewing one or two leaves. Serious fevers and malaria should be treated with drugs known to be effective in these conditions. New drugs are needed in the treatment of malaria. Perhaps vinegar weed may one day provide new compounds for the treatment of malaria. It is safe to use vinegar weed in moderation to decrease minor pain from tooth ache, stomach ache and head ache. If vinegar weed does not decrease pain, use a standard pain relieving drug. It is safe to use vinegar weed to keep insects away. This can be done by wearing a sprig of vinegar weed on a hat or necklace. The disinfectant properties of vinegar weed are not known. It is best to use a product that is known to have adequate disinfectant properties. Bleeding from the nose or uterus is best treated with standard therapies, rather than vinegar weed that has not been tested for its coagulant properties.

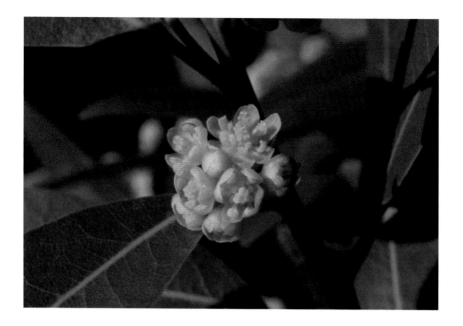

Scientific name – Umbellularia californica
Common names – California bay, California laurel, pepperwood,
psha'n (pronounced pshakn, Chumash)

Identification – This plant grows as a large, evergreen tree, up
to 130 feet high. The bark can be greenish or red-brown. The
leaves are oblong, shiny, smooth, deep green and up to 4 inches
long. The flowers are light yellow and grow in umbels. The fruit
is spherical, about three quarters of an inch in diameter, and
resembles a small, green olive (1).

Characteristics – This tree grows in ravines usually near
permanent water and can be found from 1,000 to 5,000 feet in
elevation (1). The plant has a very strong smell of bay. The leaves
have a pungent, soothing flavor when placed in the mouth. When
a dried or fresh leaf is chewed, the flavor is very intense and
peppery, hot like black pepper corns.

Distribution – California bay is found from Oregon to California (1).
In Oregon, it is called Oregon myrtle.

Primary uses – California bay was used to relieve toothache pain, simply by chewing the leaves. Tooth and gum diseases were a problem among California Indians, as discussed under Carrizo cane. The leaves were also used to repel insects. Louse and flea infestations occurred among California Indians. A tea was made from the leaves to cure diarrhea, even dysentery (4).

"California bay is an immunity enhancer. It was eaten the first couple of weeks at the start of the season to enhance immunity. Today people use it for migraine. Use sixteen leaves that have to be torn apart and deveined. Once they are deveined and put in a cloth, they open up the breathing passages and relieve any kind of edgey pain in the head." Cecilia Garcia (Chumash)

"I have suffered from migraine head aches my whole life. I have tried every migraine medication available. California bay is the only thing that gives me relief from my migraines. I put a leaf in my mouth and hold it there until the migraine is gone, within ten minutes or so." Denice Garcia (Chumash)

Secondary uses – California bay was used for aroma therapy in the hot springs around Southern California. People bathed in the California bay leaf steeped, hot springs to relieve arthritis pain. The hot springs were considered sacred and were blessed with prayers and the red flowers of Calandrinia ciliata, khutash (15). The Salinan used a poultice of the leaves to cure insanity. The smoke from burning leaves was used as an insecticide and to treat colds. California bay leaf tea was used for colds, to wash sores, and for menstrual cramps. The seeds and fruit pods were eaten as food. California bay leaves can be used to flavor foods just like commercial bay leaves, but have a stronger flavor (4).

Active compounds – California bay contains many active compounds including cineole, thujene, umbellulone, sabinene and flavonoids (263). Sabinene has a smell of pine. Cineole smells like eucalyptus. Thujene smells like soy sauce and grass. There are probably many active compounds yet to be identified from this plant.

Recommendations – Aroma therapy with California bay is pleasant and recommended. However, some people complain of head aches from this aroma therapy, whereas other people claim that it relieves head aches. California bay leaves can be safely used as insect repellants. A tea made from the leaves can be used in moderation to treat diarrhea, menstrual cramps and colds. The leaves, fruit pods and kernels can be eaten safely, in moderation. Insanity is a serious illness that should be treated by a health care provider. It is safe to chew on a California bay leaf to relieve tooth ache pain. Pain relief lasts for nearly half an hour. It is safe to use California bay as an immunity enhancer, simply be eating it as a spice in foods near the times when the seasons change.

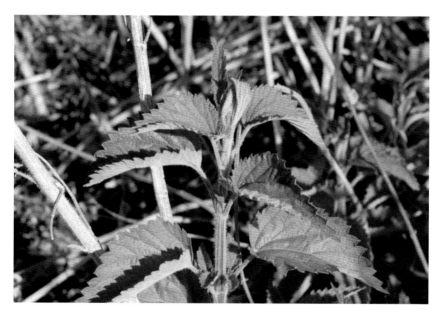

Scientific name – Urtica dioica
Common names – stinging nettle, xwhpsh (pronounced kwhapsh, Chumash)

Identification – This plant is usually about three feet tall but can grow to nine feet tall. The stems and undersides of the leaves are usually covered with stinging hairs. The leaves are usually about five inches long, grow opposite each other and are ovate. The flowers are very small and grow in racemes from the top of the plant and from the leaf petioles (1).

Characteristics – Stinging nettle is found along drainage ditches and in deep canyons. It is found below 9,000 feet in elevation (1). Stinging nettle is less common than dwarf nettle, Urtica urens, from Europe.

Distribution – This plant is found throughout North America and Northern Mexico (1).

Primary uses – Stinging nettle was used throughout Southern California to relieve arthritis pain. The stems were struck against the painful area of the body (4). This results in extreme discomfort from stinging that lasts for about 20 minutes. After this, there is a relief from pain that can last for hours or days.

Secondary uses – The leaves were brewed into a tea to treat colds and pains. The roots were made into a tea to treat dysmenorrhea and tuberculosis. The leaves were also boiled and eaten as food (4).

Active compounds – The stinging trichomes of stinging nettle contain many active compounds such as histamine, serotonin, choline, leukotrienes and other compounds (3). These compounds may alter pain perception. The leaves contain several flavonoids such as quercitin, kempferol and rhamnetin (3). Triterpenes and sterols are also present. Extracts of the leaves have been shown to have anti-inflammatory activity and to stimulate urination (3). One of the anti-inflammatory compounds in the leaves has been identified as caffeic malic acid (264). The roots contain an anti-inflammatory polysaccharide (265).

Recommendations – Stinging nettle has been tested in clinical trials and is approved for use in arthritis in Germany (3). It is safe, but initially painful to use the sting from stinging nettle for arthritis pain relief. It is safe to eat boiled nettle leaf as a food and for possible relief of arthritis pain. The taste is mild and pleasant. It is safe to use a leaf tea, in moderation, for colds and pains. A root tea can be safely used in the treatment of dysmenorrhea. However, dysmenorrhea should also be treated with a known anti-inflammatory agent. Tuberculosis should be treated with agents known to be effective, not stinging nettle. However, it may be safe to add stinging nettle therapy to standard tuberculosis therapy, provided that you discuss this addition with your health care provider. Stinging nettle root extracts have been tested in clinical trails and are approved for use in benign prostatic hypertrophy in Germany (3). These extracts have been shown to increase urination. Stinging nettle is used in combination with saw palmetto for benign prostatic hypertrophy.

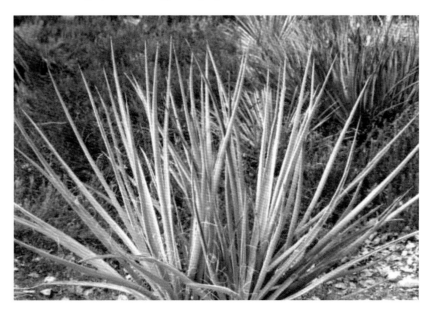

Scientific name – Yucca baccata
Common names – Spanish bayonet

Identification – This plant grows as a dense clump of basal leaves. The leaves are green, flat, up to two and a half feet long and about two inches wide. The leaf margins tend to shred leaving fibers hanging. The flower stalk is about six feet tall. The flowers form in a panicle, are bell shaped, brown on the outside and about two inches wide. The fruit is a large capsule about six inches long (1).

Characteristics – Spanish bayonet is an uncommon plant found in Joshua tree areas of some desert mountains. It is found from 2,400 to 4,000 feet in elevation (1). The name Spanish bayonet may come from a battle in which California Indians near San Diego surprised the Spanish and won the battle by using the flower stalks of yucca plants (perhaps Yucca whipplei) as bayonets.

Distribution – This plant is found in the desert mountains of California and east to Utah and Texas (1).

Primary uses – The roots of Spanish bayonet were used to make soap. The Cahuilla considered this the best soap (4).

Secondary uses – The roots were used by Salinan people to treat heat stroke and as a poultice on the eyes for blindness and cataracts (4). The fruit were eaten raw or roasted. The roasted fruit was also dried into cakes for later use (4, 12).

Active compounds – Yucca plants contain saponins that are good detergents and perhaps laxatives (266).

Recommendations – It is safe to use this plant as a soap. However, this plant is uncommon in California and should not be harvested unless it is grown in your own yard. It is not safe to use the roots of this plant to treat heat stroke. People with heat stroke should be cooled by applying cool water to the skin, giving them cool water to drink, allowing them to rest in the shade and getting them to a health care provider. It is not safe to apply a poultice of this plant to the eyes. The saponins in the plant would be very irritating to the eyes. It is safe to eat the fruit of Spanish bayonet, in moderation. The fruit has been a highly sought food and gives the plant another common name, banana yucca.

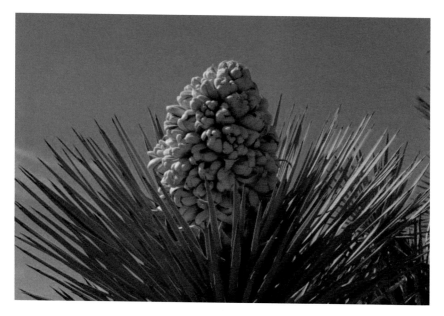

Scientific name – Yucca brevifolia
Common name – Joshua tree

Identification – These trees are very prominent on the desert and grow up to 45 feet tall. The branches are tipped with clumps of green leaves. The leaves are just over a foot long, flat and about two inches wide. The branches and trunk are densely covered with dead leaves. Flowers form at the end of the branches on a stalk that is about a foot long. The flowers form in a panicle, are cream colored and about two and a half inches wide. The flowers are seen in the early Spring from February to March. The fruit is a capsule (1).

Characteristics – Joshua trees are found in the Mojave Desert and neighboring mountains up to 6,000 feet in elevation (1).

Distribution – This plant is found in California, Nevada, Utah and Arizona (1).

Primary uses – Fibers were obtained from the leaves that were used for nets and other purposes (4).

Secondary uses – The flowers were roasted over a fire and eaten as a sweet treat (4). The pods were eaten after roasting in a stone oven, see Yucca whipplei.

Active compounds – Yucca species contain saponins (266). However, the saponins in Joshua trees do not seem to have been used medicinally.

Recommendations – It is safe to use the fibers from yucca plants to hold casts or splints in place. It is safe and apparently very desirable to eat the flowers and pods of Joshua trees. However, Joshua trees are protected in most areas of California and should not be used unless it is grown on your own property.

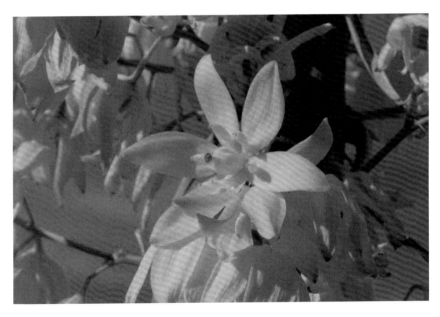

Scientific name – Yucca whipplei
Common names – Our Lord's candle,

Identification – This plant is normally made up of a dense clump of basal leaves. The leaves are tipped with a very sharp point and can be up to three feet long. The leaves are green, flat and about two inches wide at the base. At maturity, the plant sends up a long flower stalk that can be up to twelve feet high. The flowers form in a panicle, are white and about an inch and a half wide. There are six stamens and six petals. The flowers form from March to May. The fruit forms as a capsule about two inches long (1).

Characteristics – Our Lord's candle dies after flowering. The pollination of all yucca species is carried out mostly by the yucca moth, a small whitish moth. The plant is found throughout Southern California and is very common in the chaparral below 7,000 feet in elevation (1). It is also very fire resistant. The heart of the plant does not burn and quickly sends out new leaves after a fire.

Distribution – This plant is found in Southern and Baja California (1).

Primary uses – The roots of our Lord's candle were used to make soap. The flower stalks were pounded to make a laxative liquid (4). The fibers from the leaves were the strongest cordage available. The fibers were used for many purposes such as to sew the planks of Chumash canoes together, for ceremonial regalia as well as holding casts together (69). The needles on the ends of the leaves were used for sewing, sometimes with the natural cordage attached.

"Once it starts flowering, you know the weather's going to be okay. The storms are over when the yucca starts flowering." Cecilia Garcia (Chumash)

Secondary uses – Kumeyaay people used the seeds of this plant as a medication for skin irritations (4). Every Spring just before the flower stalks started to form, the hearts of this plant were collected and roasted in the ground in stone lined ovens for several days. These hearts were a very important food to many California Indians. The ovens were made by digging a long trench, lining it with stones and building a fire in the oven. Once the stones were hot, the plants were placed in the oven, protected with a layer of wet grass and covered with soil. After 24 hours, the plants were removed and eaten. The flavor was described by the Spanish explorer, Fages in 1775 as juicy and sweet with a wine like flavor (69). Apparently wine was made from yucca hearts. The leaves were used to make sandals for foot protection (4).

Active compounds – Yucca plants contain a wide variety of saponins that are very useful as detergents and perhaps as laxatives (266).

Recommendations – It is safe to use our Lord's candle as a soap to wash the hair, skin and skin irritations. It is funny that the Spanish imported cattle to raise at the Missions. Tallow was made from the cows to use for making soap and candles. If the Spanish had paid attention to the Indians, they could have had a much better soap from our Lord's candle. As a laxative, it is probably best to use the juice from the stalks as an enema, to avoid saponin toxicity. The fiber from yucca plants is very useful for holding bandages, splints and casts in place. It is safe to eat our Lord's candle after proper baking in a stone lined oven in the ground. It is safe to drink wine made from our Lord's candle, in moderation. Sandals made from this plant make good foot protection.

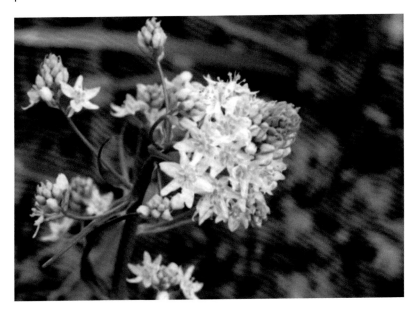

Scientific name – Zigadenus fremontii
Common name – Death camas

Identification – This plant grows to usually about ten inches tall, but can be up to two and a half feet tall. The leaves are linear and basal. They are about eight inches long and a third of an inch wide. The flowers grow in a panicle of many flowers. The flowers are about three quarters of an inch wide, are made of six perianth parts that look like petals and are white. There are two green, yellow glands at the base of each perianth part (1).

Characteristics – Death camas is found in grassy or wooded canyons where it tends to grow in the shade of other plants. It is found below 3,000 feet in elevation (1). It grows must abundantly in the year after a fire.

Distribution – This plant is found from Oregon to Baja California (1).

Primary uses – A poultice was made from many Zigadenus species for sprains, swellings, bruises and arthritis pain. Even burns and snake bites were poulticed with death camas (4).

Secondary uses – Some Zigadenus species were used as food. The bulbs were dried, and submerged in streams for three days before cooking and eating (4). This is a dangerous practice that nearly killed several men on the Lewis and Clark expedition.

Active compounds – There have been no investigations of the compounds in Zigadenus plants. Toxicity from eating improperly prepared Zigadenus bulbs is low blood pressure and low heart rate, that can lead to death (267).

Recommendations – It is probably safe to use a poultice of death camas for treating sprains, swellings, bruises and minor burns. Sprains and swellings are best treated with rest, ice, compression and elevation. Arthritis should be treated with anti-inflammatory drugs that can slow down the progression of the disease. Poisonous snake bites should be treated in the hospital with antivenom. It is not recommended to eat or take internally any preparation of death camas.

Sacred not Psychedelic

In California, Datura wrightii, Nicotiana various species, Pogonomyrmex californicus, Thamnosma montana and other species have been used to induce sacred dreams. These dreams are the way to God, in other words a powerful form of prayer. Religious freedom laws protect the use of these species in worship.

Prayer provides comfort that is vital in healing. Prayer, in the form of meditation also helps people control anxiety disorders, autoimmune illness, blood pressure, chronic and acute pain, diabetes, emotional disturbances, epilepsy, fibromyalgia, heart disease, hypertension, insomnia, cancer and premenstrual syndrome, as demonstrated in several clinical trials (268-275). Prayer has been shown to be safe in hospital settings (276). Many people believe that prayer or sacred plants provide spiritual experiences that help them heal.

Spiritual experiences can be measured scientifically. For instance, a sacred plant, such as peyote or psilocybe mushrooms, can be given to a group of people to induce spiritual experiences in the form of sacred dreams. The effects of these spiritual experiences can then be measured in each person (277), such as by measuring charitability, hours spent volunteering to help others and positive changes in personality.

Spiritual experiences and chemicals from sacred plants stimulate the spiritual sense. The spiritual sense gives us many feelings such as conscience, right and wrong, good and bad, comfort, inspiration, creativity and compassion. The spiritual sense is recognized by many religions around the world. Christianity teaches us that we have the Holy Spirit within us. Hindus believe that Brahman is present in our hearts. In Buddhism, compassion and the sense of right and wrong are essential to existence.

Many sacred species can be used to induce sacred dreams including peyote, psilocybe mushrooms, sacred Datura, tobacco, harvester ants, Salvia divinorum, morning glory seeds, ayahuasca and ibogaine. Kinetic activities such as the whirling dervishes and running also induce sacred dreams. These stimuli use a variety of chemicals to induce sacred dreams.

Chemicals that invoke sacred dreams include mescaline, psilocybin, scopolamine, nicotine, nicotinic kinins, salvinorin A, ergine, N,N-dimethyltryptamine, ibogaine, enkephalins and endorphins. All of these chemicals come from the sacred species and activities in the paragraph above. Each of these chemicals binds to specific receptors found on neurons in the brain. Binding to these receptors causes changes in the neurons that brings about a sacred dream. The receptors that bind to these chemicals are serotonin (5-HT2A/C) receptors (278), muscarinic receptors (279), nicotinic receptors (280) and opioid receptors (281). There are several chemicals and receptors that all invoke sacred dreams. How does this happen?

All of the sacred chemicals interact with receptors that alter the activity of pyramidal neurons in layer 5 of the cerebral cortex. Pyramidal neurons are part of the learning and memory system. They use either gamma-aminobutyric acid (GABA) or glutamic acid as neurotransmitters. They have a huge array of dendrites that form synapses with many other neurons. Some of these synapses have serotonergic (278), muscarinic (279), nicotinic (280) or opioid receptors (281) that mediate synaptic transmission. By binding to these receptors and altering the activity of pyramidal neurons, each of the sacred chemicals induces sacred dreams. Therefore, pyramidal neurons in layer 5 of the cerebral cortex are the source of the spiritual sense.

In Chumash society, people use sacred species to invoke sacred dreams perhaps four times during their lives. These sacred dreams are sought to help people accept more responsibility. Sacred dreams are not escapes from reality. The first sacred dream helps a child begin the journey to adulthood. The second sacred dream helps a person accept a spouse. The third sacred dream helps a person accept becoming a parent. The final sacred dream helps a person accept the responsibility of death.

The first sacred dream is a challenge that not all children survive. The child must be willing to accept the responsibility of becoming an adult in order to survive. The child is prepared a year in advance for the momoy experience. The first day of the ceremony involves preparing the child to sleep, with the singing of lullabies. The mother gives the sacred preparation to the child. A fire is started and must be kept lit at all times during the four day ceremony. The healers stand vigil as the child begins the sacred dream, that may last for two days. The third day is a time of counseling as the healers help the person recover. The fourth day is the time the healers help the person interpret their dreams. The community welcomes the person into the journey to adulthood. The person accepts a profession. When the person learns the profession, the person earns a place in the village.

The second, third and fourth sacred dreams are milder experiences. Milder preparations are used such that the sacred dreams are shorter. The person has already earned a place in the village and does not need to be challenged again.

All sacred dreams have dangers. Mescaline and psilocybin cause vomiting that may lead to lung damage if vomit is inhaled. Scopolamine causes respiratory depression. Nicotine causes vomiting and seizures. Salvinorin A and other opioid receptor binding compounds cause respiratory depression and seizures. Sacred dreams should be used appropriately and under the care of a healer experienced with the preparation.

Our society has very few healers trained in the proper use of sacred species. Young people experiment with sacred plants as an escape from reality, which is not appropriate. When these young people get into medical trouble or die, public outrage is turned onto the sacred plants. This has lead to the outlawing of some sacred plants. All of these sacred species are protected by religious freedom laws and should not be outlawed. What our society needs are healers who can supervise the proper use of sacred species. When we learn to properly use sacred dreams, we can develop the spiritual maturity that will help us function as responsible members of society.

References
1. Hickman, JC. The Jepson manual of higher plants of California. University of California Press, Berkeley, 1996.
2. Niehaus, TF and Ripper, CL. Peterson field guides Pacific States wildflowers. Houghton Mifflin Co, Boston, 1976.
3. Bisset NG. Herbal drugs and phytopharmaceuticals. CRC Press,

Boca Raton, 1994.
4. Strike SS. Ethnobotany of the California Indians, vol 2 aboriginal uses of California's indigenous plants. Koeltz Scientific Books USA, Champaign, 1994.
5. Proksch, M, Weissenboeck, G, Rodriguez, E. Flavonoids and phenolic acides in Adenostoma. Phytochem 24: 2889-2892 (1985).
6. Williams MC, Olsen JD. Toxicity of seeds of three Aesculus spp to chicks and hamsters. Am J Vet Res 45: 539-42 (1984).
7. Bhatt JP. Neurodepressive action of a piscicidal glycoside of plant, Aesulus indica (Colebr.) in fish. Indian J Exp Biol 30: 437-9 (1992).
8. Konoshima T, Lee KH. Antitumor agents, 82. Cytotoxic sapogenols from Aesculus hippocastanum. J Nat Prod 49: 650-6 (1986).
9. Sirtori CR. Aescin: pharmacology, pharmacokinetics and therapeutic profile. Pharmacol Res 44: 183-93 (2001).
10. Takegoshi K, Tohyama T, Okuda K, Suzuki K, Ohta G. A case of venoplant induced hepatic injury. Gastroent Jap 21: 62-5 (1986).
11. Yoshikawa M, Murakami T, Matsuda H, Yamahara J, Murakami N, Kitagawa I. Bioactive saponins and glycosides III. Horse chestnut (1) the structures, inhibitory effects on ethanol absorption and hypoglycemic activity of escins Ia, Ib, IIa, IIb and IIIa from the seeds of Aesculus hippocastanum. Chem Pharm Bull 44: 1454-64 (1996).
12. Cornett JW. How Indians used desert plants. Natural Trails Press, Palm Springs, 2002.
13. Abdel-Khalik SM, Miyase T, Melek FR, el-Shabraway OA, Mahmoud II, Mina SA. New steroidal saponins from Agave lophanthe Schiede and their pharmacological evaluation. Pharamazie 57: 562-6 (2002).
14. Ricks MR, Vogel PS, Elston DM, Hivnor C. Purpuric agave dermatitis. J Am Acad Dermatol 40: 356-8 (1999).
15. Walker PL, Hudson T. Chumash healing changing health and medical practices in an American Indian society. Malki Museum Press, Banning, 1993.
16. Weyrauch R. Herbal remedies. Solstice J 1: 1-27 (1982).
17. Timbrook J. Virtuous herbs: plants in Chumash medicine. J Ethnobiol 7: 171-180 (1987).
18. Acharya RN, Chaubal MG. Essential oil of Anemopsis californica. J Pharm Sci 57: 1020- 791 (1968).
19. Sanvordeker DR, Chaubal MG. Essential oil of Anemopsis californica part II, minor constituents. J Pharm .Sci 58: 1213-1217 (1969).
20. Chen M, Liu F. Sedative chemical constituents of leaves of Apocynum venetum Linn. Zhongguo Zhong Yao Za Zhi 16: 609-11 (1991).
21. Butterweck V, Nishibe S, Sasaki T, Uchida M. Antidepressant effects of Apocynum venetum leaves in a forced swimming test. Biol Pharm Bull 24: 848-51 (2001).
22. Xiong Q, Fan W, Tezuka Y, Adnyana IK, Stampoulis P, Hattori M, Namba T, Kadota S. Hepatoprotective effect of Apocynum venetum

Healing with medicinal plants by Garcia and Adams

and its active constituents. Planta Med 66: 127-33 (2000).
23. Abe F. Yamauchi T. Cardenolide glycosides from the roots of Apocynum cannabinum. Chem Pharm Bull 42: 2028-31 (1994).
24. Chen SB, Gao GY, Leung HW, Yeung HW, Yan JS, Xiao PG. Aquiledine and isoaquiledine, novel flavonoid alkaloids from Aquilegia ecalcarata. J Nat Prod 64: 85-87 (2001).
25. Bylka W. Flavonoids in the leaves with stems of some species of the Aquilegia L genus. Acta Pol Pharm 59: 57-60 (2002).
26. Yoshimitsu H, Nishidas M, Hashimoto R, Nohara T. Cycloartane type glycosides from Aquilegia flabellata. Phytochem 51: 449-52 (1999).
27. Bean LJ, Saubel KS. Temalpakh Cahuilla Indian knowledge and usage of plants. Malki Museum Press, Morongo Indian Reservation, 1972.
28. Geissman TA, Griffin TS, Irwin MA. Sesquiterpene lactones of Artemisia. Artecalin from A. californica and A tripartite ssp rupicola. Phytochem 8: 1297-1300 (1969).
29. Van Allen Murphy E. Indian uses of native plants. Mendocino County Historical Society, Fort Bragg, 1959.
30. Mead GR. The ethnobotany of the California Indians a compendium of the plants, their users and their uses. Museum of Anthropology, Greeley, 1972.
31. Brown D, Asplund RO, McMahon VA. Phenolic constituents of Artemisia tridentata spp vaseyana. Phytochem 14: 1083-4 (1975).
32. Gunawardena K, Rivera SB, Epstein WW. The monoterpenes of Artemisia tridentate ssp vaseyana, Artemisia cana ssp viscidula and Artemisia tridentate ssp spiciformis. Phytochem 59: 197-203 (2002).
33. Asplund RO, McKee M, Balasubramaniyan P. Artevasin: a new sesquiterpene lactone from Artemisia tridentata. Phytochem 11: 3542-44 (1972).
34. Evans WC. Trease and Evans Pharmacognosy. WB Sauders, Edinburgh, 2002.
35. Sikorska M, Matlawska I. Kaempferol, isorhamnetin and their glycosides from the flowers of Asclepias syriaca. Acta Polon Pharm 58: 269-72 (2001).
36. Abe F, Mori Y, Okabe H, Yamauchi T. Steroidal constituents from the roots and stems of Asclepias fruticosa. Chem Pharm Bull 42: 1777-83 (1994).
37. Abe F, Yamauchi T. 5,11-Epoxymegastigmanes from the leaves of Asclepias fruticosa. Chem Pharm Bull 48: 1908-11 (2000).
38. Sikorska M, Matlawska I, Glowniak K, Zgorka G. Qualitative and quantitative analysis of phenolic acids in Asclepias syriaca. Acta Polon Pharm 57: 69-72 (2000).
39. Haribal M, Renwick JA. Oviposition stimulants for the monarch butterfly: flavonol glycosides from Asclepias curassavica. Phytochem 41: 139-44 (1996).

40. Bedir E, Pugh N, Calis I, Pasco DS, Khan IA. Immunostimulatory effects of cycloartane-type triterpene glycosides from astagalus species. Biol Pharm Bull 23: 834-7 (2000).
41. Stegelmeier BL, James LF, Panter KE, Ralphs MH, Gardner DR, Molyneux RJ, Pfister JA. The pathogenesis and toxicokinetics of locoweed (Astragalus and Oxytropis spp) poisoning in livestock. J Nat Toxins 8: 35-45 (1999).
42. Keckeis K, Sarker SD, Dinan LN. Phytoecdysteroids from Atriplex nummularia. Fitoter 71: 456-8 (2000).
43. Cobos MI, Rodriquez JL, Oliva ML, Demo M, Faillaci SM, Zygadlo JA. Composition and antimicrobial activity of the essential oil of Baccharis notosergila. Planta Med 67: 84-6 (2001).
44. Wachter GA, Montenegro G, Timmermann BN. Diterpenoids from Baccharis pingraea. J Nat Prod 62: 307-8 (1999).
45. Rahalison L, Benathan M, Monod M, Frenk E, Gupta MP, Solis PN, Fuzzati N, Hostettmann K. Antifungal principles of Baccharis pedunculata. Planta Med 61: 360-2 (1995).
46. Fullas F, Hussain RA, Chai HB, Pezzuto JM, Soejarto DD, Kinghorn AD. Cytotoxic constituents of Baccharis gaudichaudiana. J Nat Prod 57: 801-7 (1994).
47. Jarvis BB, Wang S, Cox C, Rao MM, Philip V, Varaschin MS, Barros CS. Brazilian Baccharis toxins: livestock poisoning and the isolation of macrocyclic trichothecene glucosides. Nat Toxins 4: 58-71 (1996).
48. Cifuente DA, Simirgiotis MJ, Favier LS, Rotelli AE, Pelzer LE. Antiinflammatory activity from aerial parts of Baccharis medullosa, Baccharis rufescens and Laennecia sophiifolia in mice. Phytother Res 15: 529-31 (2001).
49. Fukuda K, Hibiya Y, Mutoh M, Koshiji M, Akao S, Fujiwara H. Inhibition by berberine of cyclooxygenase 2 transcriptional activity in human colon cancer cells. J Ethnopharmacol 66: 227-33 (1999).
50. Shamsa F, Ahmadiani A, Khosrokhavar R. Antihistaminic and anticholinergic activity of barberry fruit (Berberis vulgaris) in the guinea pig ileum. J Ethnopharmacol 64: 161-6 (1999).
51. Stermitz FR, Lorenz P, Tawara JN, Zenewicz IA, Lewis K. Synergy in a medicinal plant: antimicrobial action of berberine potentiated by 5'-methoxyhydnocarpin, a multidrug pump inhibitor. Proc Nat Acad Sci USA 97: 1433-7 (2000).
52. Angerhofer CK, Guinaudeau H. Wongpanich V, Pezzuto JM, Cordell GA. Antiplasmodial and cytotoxic activity of natural bisbenzylisoquinoline alkaloids. J Nat Prod 62: 59-66 (1999).
53. Artschwager Kay, M. Healing with plants in the American and Mexican west. University of Arizona Press, Tucson, 1996.
54. Syamasundar KV, Mallavarapu GR. Two triterpenoid lactones from the resin of Bersera delpechiana. Phytochem 40: 337-9 (1995).
55. Souza MP, Machada MIL, Braz-Filho R. Six flavonoids from Bursera

leptophloeos. Phytochem 28: 24677-70 (1989).

56. Sosa S, Balick MJ, Arvigo R, Esposito RG, Pizza C, Altinier G, Tubaro A. Screening of the topical anti-inflammatory activity of some Central American plants. J Ethnopharmacol 81: 211-5 (2002).

57. Jolad SD, Wiedhopf, Cole JR. Cytotoxic agents from Bursera klugii (Burseraceae) I: isolation of sapelins A and B. J Pharm Sci 66: 889-90 (1977).

58. Wickramaratne DB, Mar W, Chai H, Castillo JJ, Farnsworth NR, Soejarto DD, Cordell GA, Pezzuto JM, Kinghorn AD. Cytotoxic constituents of Bursera permollis. Planta Med 61: 80-1 (1995).

59. Huacuja RL, Delgado NM, Carranco LA, Reyes LR, Rosado GA. Agglutinating and immobilizing activity of an ethanol extract of Bursera fagaroides on human and other mammalian spermatozoa. Arch Invest Med (Mex.) 21: 393-8 (1990).

60. Shakrokh R. Traditional processing of red maids, Calandrinia ciliata. The 18th California Indian Conference, Watsonville, 2003.

61. Timbrook J. Ethnobotany of Chumash Indians, California, based on collections by John P. Harrington. Econ Bot 44: 236-53 (1990).

62. Pichon-Prum N, Raynaud J, Mure C, Reynaud J. Flavonic heterosides of Ceanothus americanus L, Rhamnaceae (French). Ann Pharmaceut Francaises 43: 27-30 (1985).

63. Klein FK, Rapoport H. Ceanothus alkaloids, americine. JACS 90: 23980404 (1968).

64. Tschesche R, Frohberg E, Fehlhaber HW. Alkaloids from Rhamanaceae IV integerrin, an additional peptide alkaloid from Ceanothus integgerrimus Hock and Arn (German). Tet Lett 11: 1311-5 (1968).

65. Tschesche R, Rheingans J, Fehlhaber HW, Legler G. Integerressin and integerrenin, two peptide alkaloids from Ceanothus integerrimus Hook and Arn (German). Chem Ber 100: 3924-36 (1967).

66. Li XC, Lining C, Wu CD. Antimicrobial compounds from Ceanothus americanus against oral pathogens. Phytochem 46: 97-102 (1997).

67. Nicol H, Jacobson MB, Wallach B, Nimick J, DeJane S. Torrey Pines state reserve docent guide to plant uses. (1999).

68. Mahato SB, Ganguly AN, Sahu NP. Steroid saponins. Phytochem 21: 959-978 (1982).

69. King C. Native American Indian cultural sites in the Santa Monica Mountains. Santa Monica Mountains National Recreational Area, Thousand Oaks, 2000.

70. Schelstraete M, Kennedy BM. Composition of miner's lettuce (Montia perfoliata). J Am Diet Assoc 77: 21-5 (1980).

71. Doyle JJ. Flavonoid races of Claytonia viginica (Portulacaceae). Am J Bot 70: 1085-91 (1983).

72. Blackburn TC. December's child a book of Chumash oral narratives. University of California Press, Berkeley, 1975.

73. Shao B, Qin G, Xu R, Wu H, Ma K. Triterpenoid saponins from Clematis chinensis. Phytochem 38: 1473-9 (1995).
74. Xu R, Zhao W, Xu J, Shao B, Qin G. Studies on bioactive saponins from Chinese medicinal plants. Adv Exp Med Biol 404: 371-82 (1996).
75. Nicholls KW, Bohm BA. Flavonoids and affinities of Coreopsis bigelovii. Phytochem 18: 1076 (1979).
76. Maldonado E, Ramirez Apan MT, Perez-Castorena AL. Antiinflammatory activity of phenyl propanoids from Coreopsis mutica var mutica. Planta Med 64: 660-1 (1998).
77. Kawazu K, Nishii Y, Ishii K, Tada M. A convenient screening method for nematocidal activity. Ag Biol Chem 44: 631-6 (1980).
78. Nabhan GP. Gathering the desert. University of Arizona Press, Tucson, 1985.
79. Moerman DE. Native American ethnobotany. Timber Press, Portland, 1998.
80. Duncan KLK, Duncan MD, Alley MC, Sausville EA. Cucurbitacin E induced distuption of the actin and vimentin cytoskeleton in prostate carcinoma cells. Biochem Pharmacol 52: 1553-60 (1996).
81. Acosta Patino JL, Jimenez Balderas E, Juarez Oropeza MA, Diaz Zagoya JC. Hypoglycemic action of Cucurbita ficifolia on type 2 diabetes patients with moderately high blood glucose levels. J Ethnopharmacol 77: 99-101 (2001).
82. Miraldi E, Masti A, Ferri S, Barni Comparini I. Distribution of hyoscyamine and scopolamine in Datura stramonium. Fitoter 72: 644-8 (2001).
83. Centers for Disease Control and Prevention. Leads from the mobidity and mortality weekly report: jimson weed poisoning Texas, New York and California 1994. JAMA 273: 532-3 (1995).
84. Pfister JA, Gardner DR, Panter KE, Manners GD, Ralphs MH, Stegelmeier BL, Schoch TK. Larkspur (Delphinium spp) poisoning in livestock. J Nat Toxins 8: 81-94 (1999).
85. Pfister JA, Panter KE, Manners GD, Cheney CD. Reversal of tall larkspur (Delphinium barbeyi) poisoning in cattle with physostigmine. Vet Human Tox 36: 511-4 (1994).
86. Inoue T, Mimaki Y, Sashida Y, Nikaido T, Ohmoto T. Steroidal saponins from the tubers of Dichelostemma multiflorum and their inhibitory activity on cyclic AMP phosphodiesterase. Phytochem 39: 1103-10 (1995).
87. Spellenberg R. The Audubon Society Field Guide to North American Wildflowers Western Region. Alfred A. Knopf, New York, 1979.
88. Bjeldanes LF, Geissman TA. Sesquiterpene lactones: constituents of an F1 hybrid Encelia farinose X Encelia californica. Phytochem 10: 1079-81 (1971).
89. Rodriguez E, Towers GHN, Mitchell JC. Biological activities of

sesquiterpene lactones. Phytochem 15: 1573-1580 (1976).
90. Wellman KF. North American Indian rock art and hallucinogenic drugs. JAMA 239: 1524-7 (1978).
91. Betz JM, Gay ML, Mossoba MM, Adams S, Portz BS. Chiral gas chromatographic determination of ephedrine type alkaloids in dietary supplements containing ma huang. J AOAC Int 80: 303-15 (1997).
92. al-Khalil S, Alkofahi A, el-Eisawi D, al-Shibib A. Transtorine, a new quinoline alkaloid from Ephedra transitoria. J Nat Prod 61: 262-3 (1998).
93. Stecher PG. The Merck Index, 8th edition. Merck and Co, Rahway, 1974.
94. Walker PL, Johnson JR. Effects of contact on the Chumash Indians. In Disease and Demography in the Americas, Verano J, Ubelaker D (Eds), Smithsonian Institution Press, Washington DC, 1992, pp 127-139.
95. Forest Service. Aliso Canyon interpretive trail brochure, Santa Ynez Recreation Area. Goleta, 1993.
96. Liu YL, Ho DK, Cassady JM, Cook VM, Baird WM. Isolation of potential cancer chemopreventive agents from Eriodictyon californicum. J Nat Prod 55: 357-63 (1992).
97. Park SU, Yu M, Facchini PJ. Antisense RNA mediated suppression of benzophenanthidine alkaloid biosynthesis in transgenic cell cultures of California poppy. Plant Physiol 128: 696-706 (2002).
98. Rolland A, Fleurentin J, Lanhers MC, Misslin R, Mortier F. Neurophysiological effects of an extract of Eschscholzia californica Cham. (Papaveraceae). Phytother Res 15: 377-81 (2001).
99. Clarke CB. Edible and useful plants of California. University of California Press, Berkeley, 1977.
100. Jensen SF, Nielsen BJ. Iridoid glucosides in Fouquieriaceae. Phytochem 21: 1623-30 (1982).
101. Dominguez XA, Velasquez JO, Guerra D. Extractives from the flowers of Fouquieria splendens. Phytochem. 11: 2888 (1972).
102. Graham JG, Quinn ML, Fabricant DS, Farnsworth NR. Plants used against cancer- an extension of the work of Jonathan Hartwell. J Ethnopharmacol 73: 347-77 (2000).
103. Lovell CR. Phytodermatitis. Clin Dermatol 15: 607-13 (1997).
104. West I. Cholera and other plagues of the gold rush. A Golden Note by the Sacramento County Historical Society 46: 1-21 (2000).
105. Castillo ED. Short overview of California Indian history. At http:// ceres.ca.gov/nahc/califindian.html.
106. Latta FF. Handbook of Yokuts Indians. Brewer's Historical Press and Coyote Press, Salinas, 1999.
107. de Champ WH, Pelletier SW. Veatchine: coexistence of epimers in a crystal structure. Science 198: 726-727 (1977).
108. Mears JA. Chemical constituents and systematics of amentiferae.

Healing with medicinal plants by Garcia and Adams

Brittonia 25: 385-94 (1973).
109. Cameron DW, Feutrill GI, Perlmutter P, Sasse JM. Iridoids of Garrya elliptica as plant growth inhibitors. Phytochem 23: 533-535 (1984).
110. Morimoto M, Kumeda S, Komai K. Insect antifeedant flavonoids from Gnaphalium affine D. Don. J Ag Food Chem 48: 1888-91 (2000).
111. Meragelman TL, Silva GL, Mongelli E, Gil RR. Ent-Pimarane type diterpenes from Gnaphalium gaudichaudianum. Phytochem 62: 569-572 (2003).
112. Villagomez-Ibarra JR, Sanchez M, Espejo O, Zumiga-Estrada A, Torres-Valencia JM, Joseph-Nathan P. Antimicrobial activity of three Mexican Gnaphalium species. Fitoter 72: 692-4 (2001).
113. Adams JD et al. Grindelia camporum. Natural Standard Research Database. Boston, MA: Natural Standard, (www.naturalstandard.com, 2007).
114. Marcia FA, Torres A, Galindo JL, Varela RM, Alvarez JA, Molinilla JM. Bioactive terpenoids from sunflower leaves. Phytochem 61: 687-92 (2002).
115. Suseelan KN, Mitra R, Pandey R, Sainis KB, Krishna TG. Purification and characterization of a lectin from wild sunflower Helianthus tuberosus tubers. Arch Biochem Biophys 407: 241-7 (2002).
116. Rao YK, Rao CV, Kishore PH, Gunasekar D. Total synthesis of heliannone A and (R,S)-heliannone B, two bioactive flavonoids from Helianthus annuus cultivars. J Nat Prod 64: 368-9 (2001).
117. Balls EK. Early uses of California plants. University of California Press, Berkeley, 1962.
118. Wilkins C. Galloyl glucose derivatives from Heuchera cylindrica. Phytochem. 27: 2317-8 (1988).
119. Murga J, Garcia-Fortanet J, Carda M, Marco JA. Stereoselective synthesis of (+)-hytolide. Tet Lett 44: 1737-9 (2003).
120. Urones JG, Marcos IS, Diez D, Cubillar L. Tricyclic diterpenes from Hyptys dilatata. Phytochem 48: 1035-8 (1998).
121. Collins DO, Ruddock PL, Chiverton de Grasse J, Reynolds WF, Reese PB. Microbial transformation of cadina-4,10(15)-dien-3-one, aromadendr-1(10)-en-9-one and methyl ursolate by Mucor plumbeus ATCC 4740. Phytochem 59: 479-88 (2002).
122. Pereds-Miranda R, Hernandez L, Villavicencio MJ, Novelo M, Ibarra P, Chai H, Pezzuto JM. Structure and stereochemistry of pectinolides A-C, novel antimicrobial and cytotoxic 5,6-dihydro-alpha-pyrones from Hyptis pectinata. J. Nat. Prod. 56: 583-93 (1993).
123. Kuhnt M. Rimpler H, Heinrich M. Lignans and other compounds from the mixe Indian medicinal plant Hytis verticillata. Phytochem 36: 485-9 (1994).
124. Williams CA, Harborne JB, Goldblatt P. Correlations between phenolic patterns and tribal classification in the family iridaceae. Phytochem 25: 2135-54 (1986).

125. Wong SM, Oshima Y, Pezzuto JM, Fong HH, Farnsworth NR. Plant anticancer agents XXXIX. Triterpenes from Iris missouriensis (iridaceae). J Pharm Sci 75: 317-20 (1986).
126. Wong SM, Pezzuto JM, Fong HH, Farnsworth NR. Isolation, structural elucidation and chemical synthesis of 2-hydroxy-3-octadecyl-5-methoxy-1,4-benzoquinone (irisoquin), a cytotoxic constituent of Iris missouriensis. J Pharm Sci 74: 1114-6 (1985).
127. Marner FJ, Horper W. Phenols and quinones from seeds of different Iris species. Helv Chim Acta 75: 1557-62 (1992).
128. Stark M. A flower watcher's guide to wildflowers of the western Mojave desert. Milt Stark, Lancaster, 2000.
129. Belzer TJ. Roadside plants of Southern California. Mountain Press Publishing Co, Missoula, 1984.
130. Griffiths DW, Deighton N, Birch ANE, Patrian B, Baur R, Stadler E. Identification of glucosinolates on the leaf suface of plants from the cruciferae and closely related species. Phytochem 57: 693-700 (2001).
131. Hyder PW, Fredrickson EL, Estell RE, Tellez M, Gibbens RP. Distribution and concentration of total phenolics, condensed tannins and nordihydroguaiaretic acid (NDGA) in creosotebush (Larrea tridentate). Biochem Systemat Ecol 30: 905-912 (2002).
132. Lambert HD, Zhao D, Meyers RO, Kuester RK, Timmermann BN, Dorr RT. Nordihydrogauiaretic acid: hepatotoxicity and detoxification in the mouse. Toxicon 40: 1701-8 (2002).
133. Ciccio JF, Soto VH, Poveda LJ. Essential oil of Lepechinia schiedeana (Lamiaceae) from Costa Rica. Rev Biol Trop 47: 373-5 (1999).
134. Eggers MD, Sinnwell V, Stahl-Biskup E. (-)-Spirolepechinene, a spirosesquiterpene from Lepechinia bullata (Lamiaceae). Phytochem. 51: 987-90 (1999).
135. Ahmed AA, Hussein NS, De Adams AA, Mabry TJ. Abietane diterpenes from Lepechinia urbaniana. Pharmazie 50: 279-80 (1995).
136. Dimayuga RE, Garcia SK, Nielsen PH, Christophersen C. Traditional medicine of Baja California Sur (Mexico). III. Carnosol: a diterpene antibiotic from Lepechinia hastata. J Ethnopharmacol 31: 43-8 (1991).
137. Dean FM, Costa A, Harborne JB, Smith DM. Leptodactylone, a yellow coumarin from Leptodactylon and Linanthus species. Phytochem 17: 505-9 (1978).
138. Burgin SG, Hunter FF. Nectar versus honeydew as sources of sugar for male and female black flies (Diptera: Simuliidae). J Med Entomol 34: 605-8 (1997).
139. Fossen R, Slimestad R, Ovstedal DO, Anderson OM. Anthocyanins of grasses. Biochem Systemat Ecol 30: 855-864 (2002).
140. Foster S, Hobbs C. Peterson field guides western medicinal plants

and herbs. Houghton Mifflin Co, New York, 2002.
141. Damaj MI, Patrick GS, Creasy KR, Martin BR. Pharmacology of lobeline a nicotinic receptor ligand. J Pharmacol Exp Ther 282: 410-9 (1997).
142. Lee TT, Kashiwada Y, Huang L, Snider J, Cosentino M, Lee KH. Suksdorfin, an anti-HIV principle from Lomatium suksdorfii, its structure activity correlation with related coumarins, and synergistic effects with anti AIDS nucleosides. Bioorg Med Chem 2: 1051-6 (1994).
143. Van Wagenen BC, Huddleston J, Cardellina JH. Native American food and medicinal plants 8. Water soluble constituents of Lomatium dissectum. J Nat Prod 51: 136-41 (1988).
144. Pothier J, Cheav SL, Galand N, Dormeau C, Viel C. A comparative study of the effects of sparteine, lupanine and lupin extract on the central nervous system of the mouse. J Pharm Pharmacol 50: 949-54 (1998).
145. Shih NJ, McDonald KA, Girbes T, Iglesias R, Kohlhoff AJ, Jackman AP. Ribosome inactivating proteins of wild Oregon cucumber (Marah oreganus). Biol Chem 379: 721-5 (1998).
146. Peumans WJ, Allen AK, Nsimba-Lubaki N, Chrispeels MJ. Related glycoprotein lectins from root stocks of wild cucumbers. Phytochem 26: 909-12 (1987).
147. MacMillan J, Ward DA, Phillips AL, Sanchez-Beltran MJ, Gaskin P, Lange T, Hedden P. Gibberellin biosynthesis from gibberellin A12-aldehyde in endosperm and embryos of Marah macrocarpus. Plant Physiol 113: 1369-77 (1997).
148. Kupchan SM, Meshulam H, Sneden AT. New cucurbitacins from Pharmium tenax and Marah oreganus. Phytochem 17: 767-9 (1978).
149. Hylands PJ, Salama AM. Maragenins I, II and III, new pentacyclic triterpenes from Marah macrocarpus. Tet 35: 417-20 (1979).
150. Sims SN, James R, Christensen T. Another death due to ingestion of Nicotiana glauca. J Forensic Sci 44: 447-9 (1999).
151. Keinanen M, Oldham NJ, Baldwin IT. Rapid HPLC screening of jasmonate induced increases in tobacco alkaloids, phenolics and diterpene glycosides in Nicotiana attenuata. J Ag Food Chem 49: 3553-8 (2001).
152. Hardman JG, Limbird LE, Gilman AG. Goodman and Gilman's the pharmacological basis of therapeutics 10th edition. McGraw Hill, New York, 2001.
153. Shukla YN, Srivastava A, Kumar S, Kumar S. Phytotoxic and antimicrobial constituents of Argyreia speciosa and Oenthera biennis. J Ethnopharmacol 67: 241-5 (1999).
154. Lorenz P, Stermitz FR. Oxindole-3-acetic acid methylester from the flowers (buds) of Oenothera species. Biochem Sytemat Ecol 28: 189-91 (2000).

155. Balasinska B. Hypocholesterolemic effect of dietary evening primrose (Oenothera paradoxa) cake extract in rats. Food Chem 63: 453-9 (1998).
156. De La Cruz JP, Martin-Romero M, Carmona JA, Villalobos MA, Sanchez de la Cuesta F. Effect of evening primrose oil on platelet aggregation in rabbits fed an atherogenic diet. Thrombosis Res 87: 141-9 (1997).
157. El Kossori RL, Villaume C, El Boustani E, Sauvaire Y, Mejean L. Composition of pulp, skin and seeds of prickly pears fruit (Opuntia ficus indica sp). Plant Foods Human Nut 52: 263-70 (1998).
158. Park EH, Kahng JH, Lee SH, Shin KH. An anti-inflammatory principle from cactus. Fitoter 72: 288-90 (2001).
159. Loro JF, del Rio I, Perez-Santana L. Preliminary studies and anti-inflammatory properties of Opuntia dillenii aqueous extract. J Ethnopharmacol 67: 213-8 (1999).
160. Fernandez ML, Lin EC, Trejo A, McNamara DJ. Prickly pear (Opuntia sp) pectin alters hepatic cholesterol metabolism without affecting cholesterol absorption in guinea pigs fed a hypercholesterolemic diet. J Nut 124: 817-24 (1994).
161. Frati-Munari AC, Gordillo BE, Altamirano P, Ariza CR. Hypoglycemic effect of Opuntia streptacantha Lemaire in NIDDM. Diabetes Care 11: 63-6 (1988).
162. Ahmad A, Davies J, Randall S, Skinner GR. Antiviral properties of extract of Opuntia streptacantha. Antiviral Res 30: 75-85 (1996).
163. Oh GS, Pae HO, Oh H, Hong SG, Kim IK, Chai KY, Yun YG, Kwon TO, Chung HT. In vitro antiproliferative effect of 1,2,3,4,6-penta-O-galloyl-D-glucose on human hepatocellular carcinoma cell line, SK-HEP-1 cells. Cancer Let 174: 17-24 (2001).
164. Cheng JT, Wang CJ, Hsu FL. Paeoniflorin reverses guanethidine induced hypotension via activation of central adenosine A1 receptors in Wistar rats. Clin Exp Pharmacol Physiol 26: 815-6 (1999).
165. Matsuda H, Ohta T, Kawaguchi A, Yoshikawa M. Bioactive constituents of Chinese natural medicines. VI. Moutan cortex (2) structures and radical scavenging effects of suffruticosides A, B, C, D and E and galloyl-oxypaeoniflorin. Chem Pharm Bull 49: 69-72 (2001).
166. Abdel-Hafez AA, Meselhy MR, Nakamura N, Hattori M, El-Gendy MA, Mahfouz NM, Mohamed TA. New paeonilactone-A adducts formed by anaerobic incubation of paeoniflorin with Lactobacillus brevis in the presence of arylthiols. Chem Pharm Bull 49: 918-20 (2001).
167. Liu JK, Ma YB, Wu DG, Lu Y, Shen ZQ, Zheng QT, Chen ZH. Paeonilide, a novel anti-PAF active monoterpenoid derived metabolite from Paeonia delavayi. Biosci Biotech Biochem 64: 1511-4 (2000).
168. Lin HC, Ding HY, Ko FN, Teng CM, Wu YC. Aggregation inhibitory activity of minor acetophenones from Paeonia species. Planta Med

65: 595-9 (1999).
169. Chng JT, Wang CJ, Hsu FL. Paeoniflorin reverses guanethidine induced hypotension via activation of central adenosine A1 receptors in Wistar rats. Clin Exp Pharmacol Physiol 26: 815-6 (1999).
170. Hsu FL, Lai CW, Cheng JT. Antihyperglycemic effects of paeoniflorin and 8-debenzoylpaeoniflorin, glucosides from the root of Paeonia lactiflora. Planta Med 63: 323-5 (1997).
171. Tomoda M, Matsumoto K, Shimizu N, Gonda R, Ohara N. Characterization of neutral and an acidic polysaccharide having immunological activities from the root of Paeonia lactiflora. Biol Pharm Bull 16: 1207-10 (1993).
172. Yang DG. Comparison of pre- and post-treatment hepatohistology with heavy dosage of Paeonia rubra on chronic active hepatitis caused liver fibrosis. Chung-Kuo Chung Hsi I Chieh Ho Tsa Chih. 14: 207-9 (1994).
173. Zhang Y. The effects of nifedipine, diltiazem and Paeonia lactiflora Pall. On atherogenesis in rabbits. Chung-Hua Hsin Hsueh Kuan Ping Tsa Chih 19: 100-3 (1991).
174. Jia YB, Tang TQ. Paeonia lactiflora injection in treating chronic cor pulmonale with pulmonary hypertension. Chung Hsi I Chieh Ho Tsa Chih 11: 199-202 (1991).
175. Rodriguez-Loaiza P, Lira-Rocha A, Ruiz de Esparza R, Jimenez-Estrada M. Compounds isolated from Penstemon eximeus. Biochem Systemat Ecol 31: 437-8 (2003).
176. Krull RE, Stermitz FR. Trans-fused iridoid glycosides from Penstemon mucronatus. Phytochem 49: 2413-5 (1998).
177. Rabea EI, Badawy ME, Stevens CV, Smagghe G, Steurbaut W. Chitosan as antimicrobial agent: applications and mode of action. Biomacromolec 4: 1457-65 (2003).
178. Piek T. Neurotoxins from venoms of the Hymenoptera- twenty five years of research in Amsterdam. Comp Biochem Physiol C 96: 223-33 (1990).
179. Astudillo LS, Juergens KS, Schmeda-Hirschmann G, Griffith GA, Holt DJ, Jenkins PR. DNA binding alkaloids from Prosopis alba. Planta Med 65: 161-2 (1999).
180. Malhotra S, Misra K. Ellagic acid 4-O-rutinoside from pods of Prosopis juliflora. Phytochem 20: 2439-2440 (1981).
181. Jacobs E, Ferreira D, Roux DG. Atropisomerism in a new class of condensed tannins based on biphenyl and o-terphenyl. Tet Lett 24: 4627-30 (1983).
182. Washburn KE, Breshears MA, Ritchey JW, Morgan SE, Streeter RN. Honey mesquite toxicosis in a goat. J Am Vet Med Assoc 220: 1837-9 (2002).
183. Habermehl GG. Plant toxins. Toxicon 34: 298 (1996).
184. Olszewska M, Wolbis M. Flavonoids from the flowers of Prunus

spinosa. Acta Pol Pharm 58: 367-72 (2001).
185. Wolbis M. Olszewska M, Wesolowski WJ. Triterpenes and sterols in the flowers and leaves of Prunus spinosa L. (Rosaceae). Acta Pol Pharm 58: 459-62 (2001).
186. Tomas-Barberan FA, Gil MI, Cremin P, Waterhouse AL, Hess-Pierce B, Kader AA. HPLC-DAD-ESIMS analysis of phenolic compounds in nectarines, peaches and plums. J Ag Food Chem 49: 4748-60 (2001).
187. Dienta F, Martinez-Gomez P, Grane N, Martin ML, Leon A, Canovas JA, Berenquer V. Relationship between cyanogenic compounds in kernels, leaves and roots of sweet and bitter kernelled almonds. J Ag Food Chem 50: 2149-52 (2002).
188. Stacewicz-Sapuntzakis M, Bowen PE, Hussain EA, Damayanti-Wood BI, Farnsworth NR. Chemical composition and potential health effects of prunes: a functional food. Crit Rev Food Sci Nutr 41: 251-86 (2001).
189. Manikumar G, Gaetano K, Wani MC, Taylor H, Hughes TJ, Warner J, McGivney R, Wall ME. Plant antimutagenic agents 5. Isolation and structure of two new isoflavones, fremontin and fremontone from Psorothamnus fremontii. J Nat Prod 52: 769-73 (1989).
190. Zhang H, Li X, Ashendel CL, Chang CJ. Bioactive compounds from Psorothamnus junceus. J Nat Prod 63: 1244-8 (2000).
191. Garg SK, Makkar HP, Nagal KB, Sharma SK, Wadhwa DR, Singh B. Oak (Quercus incana) leaf poisoning in cattle. Vet Human Tox 34: 161-4 (1992).
192. Meng Z, Zhou Y, Lu J, Sugahara K, Xu S, Kodama H. Effect of five flavonoid compounds isolated from Quercus dentata Thunb on superoxide generation in human neutrophils and phosphorylation of neutrophil proteins. Clin Chim Acta 306: 97-102 (2001).
193. Konig M, Scholz E, Hartmann R, Lehmann W, Rimpler H. Ellagitannins and complex tannins from Quercus petraea bark. J Nat Prod 57: 1411-5 (1994).
194. Cadahia E, Munoz L, Fernandez de Simon B, Garcia-Vallejo MC. Changes in low molecular weight phenolic compounds in Spanish, French and American oak woods during natural seasoning and toasting. J Agric Food Chem 49: 1790-8 (2001).
195. Sharp H, Latif Z, Bartholomew B, Thomas D, Thomas B, Sarker SD, Nash RJ. Emodin and syringaldehyde from Rhamnus pubescens (Rhamnaceae). Biochem Sytemat Ecol 29: 113-5 (2001).
196. Prasad D, Pant G, Rawat MSM, Nagatsu A. Constituents of Rhamnus virgatus (Rhamnaceae). Biochem Systemat Ecol 28: 1027-30 (2000).
197. Lin CN, Wei BL. Anthraquinone and naphthalene glycosides from Rhamnus nakaharai. Phytochem 33: 905-908 (1993).
198. Wei BL, Lu CM, Tsao LT, Wang JP, Lin CN. In vitro anti-inflammatory effects of quercetin 3-O-methyl ether and other constituents from

Rhamnus species. Planta Med 67: 745-7 (2001).
199. Lin CN, Lu CM, Lin HC, Ko FN, Teng CM. Novel antiplatelet naphthalene from Rhamnus nakaharai. J Nat Prod 58: 1934-40 (1995).
200. van Gorkom BA, de Vries EG, Karrenbeld A, Kleibeuker JH. Review article anthranoid laxatives and their potential carcinogenic effects. Aliment Pharmacol Ther 13: 443-52 (1999).
201. Masesane IB, Yeboah SO, Liebscher J, Mugge C, Abegaz BM. A bichalcone from the twigs of Rhus pyroides. Phytochem 53: 1005-8 (2000).
202. Franke K, Masaoud M, Schmidt J. Cardanols from leaves of Rhus thyrsiflora. Planta Med 67: 477-9 (2001).
203. Wang HK, Xia Y, Yang ZY, Natschke SL, Lee KH. Recent advances in the discovery and development of flavonoids and their analogues as antitumor and antiHIV agents. Adv Exp Med Biol 439: 191-225 (1998).
204. Lin YM, Anderson H, Flavin MT, Pai YH, Mata-Greenwood E, Pengsuparp T, Pezzuto JM, Schinazi RF, Hughes SH, Chen FC. In vitro anti-HIV activity of biflavonoids isolated from Rhus succedanea and Garcinia multiflora. J Nat Prod 60: 884-8 (1997).
205. Saxena G, McCutcheon AR, Farmer S, Towers GH, Hancock RE. Antimicrobial constituents of Rhus glabra. J Ethnopharmacol 42: 95-9 (1994).
206. Kuo SC, Teng CM, Lee LG, Chiu TH, Wu TS, Huang SC, Wu JB, Shieh TY, Chang RJ, Chou TC. 6-Pentadecylsalicylic acid: an antithrombin component isolated from the stem of Rhus semialata var roxburghii. Planta Med 57: 247-9 (1991).
207. Hong DH, Han SB, Lee CW, Park SH, Jeon YJ, Kim MJ, Kwak SS, Kim HM. Cytotoxicity of urushiols isolated from sap of Korean lacquer tree (Rhus vernicifera Stokes). Arch Pharmacal Res 22: 638-41 (1999).
208. Grossi C, Raymond O, Jay M. Flavonoid and enzyme polymorphisms and taxonomic organization of Rosa sections: carolinae, cinnamonomeae, pimpinellifoliae and synstylae. Biochem Systemat Ecol 26: 857-871 (1998).
209. Hashidoko Y. The phytochemistry of Rosa rugosa. Phytochem 43: 535-49 (1996).
210. Kashiwada Y, Wang HK, Nagao T, Kitanaka S, Yasuda I, Fujioka T, Yamagishi T, Cosentino LM, Kozuka M, Okabe H, Ikeshiro Y, Hu CQ, Yeh E, Lee KH. Anti-AIDS agents 30. anti-HIV activity of oleanolic acid, pomolic acid and structurally related triterpenoids. J Nat Prod 61: 1090-5 (1998).
211. Palmer E. Plants used by the Indians of the United States. Am Naturalist 12: 646-55 (1878).
212. Luis JG, Grillo TA. New diterpenes from Salvia munzii: chemical and

biogenetic aspects. Tet 49: 6277-84 (1993).
213. Masterova I, Misikova E, Sirotkova L, Vaverkova S, Ubik K. Royleanones in the roots of Salvia officinalis of domestic provenance and their antimicrobial activity. Ceska a Slovenska Farmacie 45: 242-5 (1996).
214. Baldes LJ. Salvia divinorum and the unique diterpene hallucinogen, salvinorin (divinorin) A. J Psychoactive Drugs 26: 277-83 (1994).
215. Ulubelen A, Topcu G, Johansson CB. Norditerpenoids and diterpenoids from Salvia multicaulis with antituberculous activity. J Nat Prod 60: 1275-80 (1997).
216. Chang HM, Chui KY, Tan FWL, Yang Y, Zhong ZP. Structure activity relationship of miltirone an active central benzodiazepine receptor ligand isolated from Salvia miltiorrhiza Bunge (danshen). J Med Chem 34: 1675-92 (1991).
217. Perry R. The Chumash people: materials for teachers and students. Santa Barbara Museum of History and EZ Nature Books, Santa Barbara, 1991.
218. Adams JD, Garcia C, Wall M. Salvia columbariae contains tanshinones. In press.
219. Tang MK, Ren DC, Zhang JT, Du GH. Effect of salvianolic acids from radix salviae miltiorrhizae on regional cerebral blood flow and platelet aggregation in rats. Phytomed 9: 405-9 (2002).
220. Romussi G, Ciarallo G, Bisio A, Fontana N, De Simone R, De Tommasi N, Mascolo N, Pinto L. A new diterpenoid with antispasmodic activity from Salvia cinnabarina. Planta Med 67: 153-5 (2001).
221. Ulubelen A, Oksuz S, Kolak U, Bozok-Hohansson C, Celik C, Voelter W. Antibacterial diterpenes from the roots of Salvia viridis. Planta Med 66: 458-62 (2000).
222. Kang BY, Chung SW, Kim SH, Ryu SY, Kim TS. Inhibition of interleukin-12 and interferon gamma production in immune cells by tanshinones from Salvia miltiorrhiza. Immunopharmacol 49: 355-61 (2000).
223. Benrezzouk R, Terencio MC, Ferrandiz ML, Hernandez-Perez M, Rabanal R, Alcaraz MJ. Inhibition of 5-lipoxygenase by the natural anti-inflammatory compound aethiopinone. Inflam Res 50: 96-101 (2001).
224. Baricevic D, Sosa S, Della Loggia R, Tubaro A, Simonovska B, Krasna A, Zupancic A. Topical anti-inflammatory activity of Salvia officinalis leaves the relevance of usolic acid. J Ethnopharmacol 75: 125-32 (2001).
225. Vivian B, Tal H, Inna K. The effect of sambucol a black elderberry based natural product on the production of human cytokines1. inflammatory cytokines. Eur Cytokine Network 12: 290-6 (2001).
226. Mlinaric A. Kreft S, Umek A, Strukelj B. Screening of selected plant

extracts for in vitro inhibitory activity on HIV-1 reverse transcriptase. Pharmazie 55: 75-7 (2000).
227. Gray AM, Abdel-Wahab YH, Flatt PR. The traditional plant treatment Sambucus nigra (elder) exhibits insulin like and insulin releasing actions in vitro. J Nut 130: 15-20 (2000).
228. Beaux D, Fleurentin J, Mortier F. Effect of extracts of Orthosiphon stamineus Benth, Hieracium pilosella L, Sambucus nigra L and Arctostaphylos uva-ursi (L) Spreng in rats. Phytother Res 13: 222-5 (1999).
229. Ahmadiani A, Fereidoni M, Semnanian S, Kamalinejad M, Saremi S. Antinociceptive and anti-inflammatory effects of Sambucus ebulus rhizome extract in rats. J Ethnopharmacol 61: 229-35 (1998).
230. Li H, Li J, Prasain JK, Tezuka Y, Namba T, Miyahara T, Tonami S, Seto H, Tada T, Kadota S. Antiosteoporotic activity of the stems of Sambucus sieboldiana. Biol Pharm Bull 21: 594-8 (1998).
231. Panizzi L, Flamini G, Cioni PL, Morelli I. Composition and antimicrobial properties of essential oils of four Mediterranean Lamiaceae. J Ethnopharmacol 39: 167-70 (1993).
232. Hernandez NE, Tereschuk ML, Abdala LR. Antimicrobial activity of flavonoids in medicinal plants from Tafi del Valle (Tucuman, Argentina). J Ethnopharmacol 73: 317-22 (2000).
233. Yamasaki K, Nakano M, Kawahata T, Mori H, Otake T, Ueba N, Oishi I, Inami R, Yamane M, Makamura M, Murata H, Nakanishi T. Anti-HIV-1 activity of herbs in Labiatae. Biol Pharm Bull 21: 829033 (1998).
234. Hajhashemi V, Sadraei H, Ghannadi AR, Mohseni M. Antispasmodic and anti-diarrhoeal effect of Satureja hortansis L essential oil. J Ethnopharmacol 71: 187-92 (2000).
235. Sanchez de Rojas VR, Somoza B, Ortega T, Villar AM. Isolation of vasodilatory active flavonoids from the traditional remedy Satureja obovata. Planta Med 62: 272-4 (1996).
236. Cappillino P, Kleiman R, Botti C. Composition of Chilean jojoba seeds. Indust Crop Prod 17: 177-82 (2003).
237. Elliger CA, Waiss AC, Lundin RE. Cyanomethylenecyclohexyl glucosides from Simmondsia californica. Phytochem 13: 2319-20 (1974).
238. Cokelaere M, Cauwelier B, Cokelaere K, Flo G, Houache N, Lieverns S, Van Boven M, Decuypere E. Hematological and pathological effects of 0.25% purified simmondsin in growing rats. Indust Crop Prod 12: 165-71 (2000).
239. Crawford L, Myhr B. A preliminary assessment of the toxicity and mutagenic potential of steroidal alkaloids in transgenic mice. Food Chem Tox 33: 191-4 (1995).
240. Ceha LJ, Presperin C, Young E, Allswede M, Erickson T. Anticholinergic toxicity from nightshade berry poisoning responsive to

physostigmine. J Emerg Med 15: 65-9 (1997).

241. Kartsev VG, Stepanichenko NN, Auelbekov SA. Chemical composition and pharmacological properties of plants of the genus Stachys. Chem Nat Comp 30: 645-54 (1994).

242. Miyase T, Yamamoto R, Ueno A. Betonicosides A-D and betonicolide, diterpenoids from the roots of Stachys officinalis. Chem Pharm Bull 44: 1610-3 (1996).

243. Yamamoto R, Miyase T, Ueno A. Stachyssaponins 1-VIII, new oleanane type triterpene saponins from Stachys riederi Chamisso. Chem Pharm Bull 42: 1291-6 (1994).

244. Calis I, Basaran AA, Saracoglu I, Sticher O. Iridoid and phenylpropanoid glycosides from Stachys macra. Phytochem 31: 167-70 (1992).

245. Maleki N, Garjani A, Nazemiyeh H, Nilfouroushan N, Eftekhar Sadat AT, Allameh Z, Hasannia N. Potent anti-inflammatory activities of hydroalcoholic extract from aerial parts of Stachys inflata in rats. J Ethnopharmacol 75: 213-8 (2001).

246. Skaltsa HD, Lazari DM, Chinou IB, Loukis AE. Composition and antibacterial activity of the essential oils of Stachys candida and S chrysantha from southern Greece. Planta Med 65: 255-6 (1999).

247. Philbey AW, Hawker AM, Evers JV. A neurological locomotor disorder in sheep grazing Stachys arvensis. Aust Vet J 79: 427-30 (2001).

248. Ghosh A, Misra S, Dutta AK, Choudhury A. Pentacyclic triterpenoids and sterols from seven species of mangrove. Phytochem 24: 1725-7 (1985).

249. Piattelli M, Imperato F. Betacyanins of some chenopodiaceae. Phytochem 10: 3133-4 (1971).

250. Benwahhoud M, Jouad H, Eddouks M, Lyoussi B. Hypoglycemic effect of Suaeda fruticosa in streptozotocin induced diabetic rats. J Ethnopharmacol. 76: 35-8 (2001).

251. Bennani-Kabchi N, el Bouayadi F, Kehel L, Fdhil H, Marquie G. Effect of Suaeda fruticosa aqueous extract in the hypercholesterolaemic and insulin resistant sand rat. Therapie 54: 725-30 (1999).

252. Sendra J, Janeczko Z. Beta-sitosterol and oleanolic acid in leaves of Symphoricarpos racemosus Hooker. Pol J Pharmacol Pharm 25: 607-10 (1973).

253. Szaufer M, Kowalewski Z, Phillipson JD. Chelidonine from Symphoricarpos albus. Phytochem. 17: 1446-7 (1978).

254. Astudillo L, Rodriguez JA, Schmeda-Hirschmann G. Gastroprotective activity of oleanolic acid derivatives on experimentally induced gastric lesions in rats and mice. J Pharm Pharmacol 54: 583-8 (2002).

255. Yim TK, Wu WK, Pak WF, Ko KM. Hepatoprotective action of an olenaolic acid enriched extract of Ligustrum lucidum fruits is mediated through an enhancement on hepatic glutathione regeneration capacity in mice. Phytochem Res 15: 589-92 (2001).

256. Mengoni F, Lichtner M, Battinelli L, Marzi M, Mastroianni CM, Vullo V, Mazzanti G. In vitro anti-HIV activity of oleanolic acid on infected human mononuclear cells. Planta Med 68: 111-4 (2002).

257. Kleinrok Z, Szponar J, Matuszek B, Jagiello-Wojtowicz E. Studies on the participation of the dopaminergic system in the central effects of chelidonine. Pol J Pharmacol Pharm 42: 417-24 (1990).

258. Lewis WH. Snowberry (Symphoricarpos) poisoning in children JAMA 242: 2663 (1979).

259. Chang PT, Crodell GA, Aynilian GH, Fong HH, Farnsworth NR. Alkaloids and coumarins of Thamnosma montana. Lloydia 39: 134-40 (1976).

260. Dreyer DL. Constituents of Thamnosma montana Torr and Frem. Tet 22: 2923-7 (1966).

261. Oertli EH, Rowe LD, Lovering SL, Ivie GW, Bailey EM. Phototoxic effect of Thamnosma texana (Dutchman's breeches) in sheep. Am J Vet Res 44: 1126-9 (1983).

262. Tucker AO, Maciarello MJ. The essential oil of Trichostema dichotomum. J Ess Oil Res 2: 149-50 (1990).

263. Goralka RJL, Schumaker MA, Langenheim JH. Variation in chemical and physical properties during leaf development in California bay tree (Umbellularia californica) predictions regarding palatability for deer. Biochem System Ecol 24: 93-103 (1996).

264. Obertreis B, Giller K, Teucher T, Behnke B, Schmitz H. Anti-inflammatory effect of Urtica dioica folia extract in comparison to caffeic malic acid. Arzneim Forsch 46: 52-6 (1996).

265. Wagner H, Willer F, Kreher B. Biologically active compounds from the aqueous extract of Urtica dioica. Planta Med 55: 452-4 (1989).

266. Oleszek W, Sitek M, Stochmal A, Piacente S, Pizza C, Cheeke P. Steroidal saponins of Yucca schidigera Roezl. J Ag Food Chem 49: 4392-6 (2001).

267. Heilpern KL. Zigadenus poisoning. Ann Emerg Med 25: 259-62 (1995).

268. Anderson JW, Liu C, Kryscio R. Blood pressure response to transcendental meditation: a meta-analysis. Am J Hypertens 21: 310-6 (2008).

269. Arias AJ, Steinberg K, Banga A, Trestman RL. Systematic review of the efficacy of meditation techniques as treatments for medical illnesses. J Alt Comp Med 12: 817-32 (2006).

270. Chaiopanont S. Hypoglycemic effect of sitting breathing meditation exercise on type 2 diabetes at Wat Khae Nok Primary Health Center in Nonthaburi province. J Med Assoc Thailand 91: 93-8 (2008).

271. Gardner-Nix J, Backman S, Barbati J, Grummitt J. Evaluating distance education of a mindfulness based

meditation programme for chronic pain management. J Telemed Telecare 14: 88-92 (2008).
272.   Morone NE, Greco CM, Weiner DK. Mindfulness meditation for the control of chronic low back pain in older adults: a randomized controlled pilot study. Pain 134: 310-9 (2008).
273.   Ong JC, Shapiro SL, Manber R. Combining mindfulness meditation with cognitive behavior therapy for insomnia: a treatment development study. Behav Ther 39: 171-82 (2008).
274.   Ornish, D. Dr. Dean Ornish's program for reversing heart disease. New York, Random House (1996).
275.   Sephton SE, Salmon P, Weissbecher I, Ulmer C, Floyd A, Hoover K, Studts JL. Mindfulness meditation alleviates depressive symptoms in women with fibromyalgia: results of a randomized clinical trial. Arth Rheum 57: 77-85 (2007).
276.   Astin JA, Harkness E, Ernst E. The efficacy of 'distant healing': a systematic review of randomized trials. Ann Int Med 132: 903-10 (2000).
277.   Griffiths RR, Richards WA, McCann U, Jesse R. Psilocybin can occasion mystical-type experiences having substantial and sustained personal meaning and spiritual significance. Psychopharmacol 187: 268-83 (2006).
278.   Appel JB, Callahan PM. Involvement of 5-HT receptor subtypes in the discriminative stimulus properties of mescaline. Eur J Pharmacol 159: 41-6 (1989).
279.   Dringenberg HC, Yahia N, Cirasuolo J, McKee D, Kuo MC. Neocortical activation by electrical and chemical stimulation of the rat inferior colliculus: intra-collicular mapping and neuropharmacological characterization. Exp Brain Res 154: 461-9 (2004).
280.   Alkondon M, Albuquerque EX. The nicotinic acetylcholine receptor subtypes and their function in the hippocampus and cerebral cortex. Prog Brain Res 145: 109-120 (2004).
281.   Marek GJ, Aghajanian GK. 5-Hydroxytryptamine induced excitatory postsynaptic currents in neocortical layer V pyramidal cells: suppression by u-opiate receptor activation. Neurosci 86: 485-97 (1998).

Index

221
Candlewood 100
Cardinal flower 127
Carrizo 16, 34, 39, 41, 94, 99, 126, 211
Casts 20, 22, 27, 65, 82, 104, 117, 193, 194, 217, 218, 219
Cataracts 215
Ceanothus crassifolius 57
Ceanothus integerrimus 59
Ceanothus leucodermis 61
Chafing 37
Chamise 14
Chaparral whitethorn 61
Chest pain 68, 69, 83, 84, 203
Chewing gum 16, 34, 38, 39, 40, 41, 42, 43, 101
Chia 182
Chills 109
Chinese houses 71
Chlorogalum parviflorum 62
Chlorogalum pomeridianum 64
Christmas berry 110
Clairvoyant 203
Claytonia perfoliata 66
Clematis ligusticifolia 67
Clematis pauciflora 69
Coffeeberry 165
Colds 10, 12, 15, 16, 23, 25, 32, 33, 34, 37, 46, 59, 68, 85, 94, 95,
96, 104, 105, 106, 120, 121, 123, 130, 139, 148, 159, 162, 164,
168, 169, 170, 171, 172, 173, 174, 175, 176, 178, 180, 181, 185,
189, 190, 191, 201, 203, 207, 208, 209, 211, 212, 213
Colic 173, 187, 191, 192
Collinsia heterophylla 71
Communication 180
Constipation 120, 168, 173
Coreopsis bigelovii 72
Coughs 28, 29, 69, 94, 95, 101, 107,108, 187, 198
Coyote brush 34, 47
Coyote's rope 68, 69, 70
Creeping snowberry 201
Creosote bush 121
Crimson columbine 28
Cucurbita foetidissima 73

Cuts 25, 30, 92, 139, 140, 178
Datura wrightii 44, 75, 153, 221
Death camas 219
Debility 176
Deer brush 59
Delphinium parryi 78
Dendromecon rigida 80
Dental hygiene 39, 41, 42, 43, 127
Deodorant 180, 181, 192
Depression 35, 106, 148
Desert lavender 115
Desert milkweed 40
Desert tea 84
Desert trumpet 97
Diapers 120, 193
Diarrhea 28, 29, 30, 31, 63, 65, 77, 82, 104, 113, 153, 154, 162, 164, 176, 178, 179, 181, 192, 197, 211, 212
Dichelostoma capitatum 81
Disinfectant 37, 198, 209
Diuretic 28, 29, 65, 189
Dogbane 26
Douche 207
Dreams 9, 34, 35, 36, 76, 77, 85, 86, 90, 91, 133, 134, 137, 139, 141, 153, 181, 182, 221, 222, 223
Dyes 53, 58, 109, 110, 189
Dysentery 34, 36, 153, 211
Dysmenorrhea 34, 35, 90, 96, 170, 171, 189, 190, 213
Ear ache 34, 35, 117, 139, 187, 199
Elderberry 188
Elephant tree 54
Emetic 68, 69, 79, 111, 112, 148, 166, 189
Encelia farinosa 83
Ephedra californica 84, 88, 89, 90
Ephedra nevadensis 87
Ephedra viridis 77, 86, 89
Eriodictyon crassifolium 91
Eriodictyon trichocalyx 92, 94
Eriogonum fasciculatum 95
Eriogonum inflatum 97
Eschscholzia californica 98
Estuary sea blite 200

Nicotiana attenuata 32, 33, 136
Nicotiana glauca 137, 138
Nicotiana quadrivalvis 137, 138
Nightshade 196
Ocotillo 100
Oenothera elata 141
Opuntia basilaris 143
Opuntia littoralis 144
Oregon grape 50
Oregon myrtle 210
Our Lord's candle 217
Paeonia californica 147
Pain relief 12, 13, 17, 25, 34, 35, 44, 46, 67, 68, 69, 72, 83, 84, 92, 96, 101, 111, 117, 120, 121, 125, 128, 129, 130, 133, 134, 144, 145, 146, 148, 162, 164, 166, 168, 174, 175, 178, 181, 186, 187, 189, 196, 203, 208, 209, 211, 212, 213, 220, 221
Paint 42
Papaver californicum 149
Parkinson's disease 77
Paralysis 18, 92
Parasitic worms 74, 191, 192, 204, 205
Penstemon spectabilis 151
Pepperwood 210
Perfume 32, 173, 174
Pespibata 136, 138
Phototoxicity 203
Pig nut 194
Pigment 42, 133, 134, 200
Pipes 97, 98, 139
Pitcher sage 122
Pneumonia 69, 92, 93, 106, 169, 171, 172
Pogonomyrmex californicus 6, 152, 221
Poison 18, 19, 23, 42, 43, 44, 48, 65, 77, 79, 130, 133, 164, 207
Poison oak 34, 35, 41, 47, 48, 68, 108, 148, 149, 171, 172, 191, 204, 205
Poultice 13, 18, 20, 22, 27, 32, 38, 39, 42, 43, 47, 48, 67, 68, 69, 71, 72, 85, 86, 102, 106, 117, 121, 122, 128, 129, 130, 139, 140, 144, 145, 151, 152, 166, 176, 178, 179, 211, 215, 220
Pregnancy 25, 27, 86, 91, 120, 141, 192, 197
Premenstrual syndrome 34, 35, 189, 190, 221
Prickly pear cactus 144

Satureja douglasii 190
Sedatives 60, 99
Scirpus acutus 65, 193
Scorpion stings 125
Screwbean mesquite 156
Shampoo 58, 60, 63, 64, 68, 82, 121, 122, 134, 180, 181, 189, 189, 190, 195, 207
Shaw's agave 21
Silk tassel bush 103
Simmondsia chinensis 194
Skin disorders 151
Skin infections 15, 46, 178, 205
Skunkbrush 171
Small pox 162, 163
Small soap plant 62
Snake bites 18, 19, 42, 43, 71, 72, 115, 130, 203, 204, 205, 220
Soap 20, 58, 60, 62, 63, 64, 65, 68, 74, 82, 200, 215, 218, 219
Soap plant 64
Solanum douglasii 194, 196
Sores 15, 16, 17, 23, 25, 30, 41, 55, 61, 65, 68, 69, 85, 94, 102, 111, 112, 117, 130, 131, 140, 151, 152, 157, 166, 172, 198, 201, 202, 205, 211
Sore throat 16, 17, 23, 68, 69, 102, 107, 108, 130, 131, 139, 140, 155, 174, 175, 178, 180, 181, 187, 198
Spanish bayonet 214
Spider bites 38, 39
Spirit 4, 9, 10, 32, 33, 34, 36, 97, 139, 140, 180, 181, 182, 185, 186, 221, 222, 223
Sprains 220
Stachys bullata 198
Sticky yerba santa 94
Stinging nettle 212
Stomach ache 16, 17, 28, 29, 37, 59, 60, 73, 76, 78, 79, 88, 96, 104, 111, 117, 121, 132, 133, 148, 155, 161, 164, 168, 172, 181, 185, 191, 192, 198, 202, 207, 208, 209
Strength 25, 140, 180
Stroke 86, 88, 90, 91, 183, 184
Suaeda esteroa 199
Symphoricarpos mollis 201
Sugar 16, 35, 74, 94, 112, 126, 148, 159, 164, 183, 190
Sugar bush 169, 170, 171

Virgin's bower 67
Vomiting 20, 69, 70, 74, 75, 102, 108, 112, 126, 128, 129, 138, 139, 140, 165, 166, 178, 179, 189, 202, 205, 223
Warts 144, 165, 204, 205
Wax 101, 195
Western blue flag 116
White sage 4, 11, 98, 106, 179, 187, 192
Wild cucumber 133
Wine 35, 51, 164, 189, 190, 197, 218, 219
Witch craft 128, 129
Woolly bluecurls 206
Wounds 13, 16, 17, 18, 20, 31, 32, 36, 37, 43, 46, 47, 48, 57, 65, 86, 102, 106, 108, 139, 140, 142, 144, 145, 146, 152, 157, 165, 166, 176, 179, 181
Yarrow 12
Yeast infections 49, 141, 142
Yerba buena 187
Yerba mansa 24
Yerba santa 91, 108
Yucca baccata 214
Yucca brevifolia 216
Yucca whipplei 20, 22, 63, 65, 215, 217
Zigadenus fremontii 219

Abedus Press
PO Box 8018
La Crescenta, CA 91224

Website: www.abeduspress.com

Healing with medicinal plants of the west - cultural and scientific basis for their use

by Cecilia Garcia and James Adams

To order more books -

Cost below includes one book, tax and shipping.

Cost of one book in California: $20.33

Cost of one book outside California: $18.95

Also available from Abedus Press -

Estanislao - Warrior, Man of God

This historical novel is the story of the real Zorro. Estanislao was a Yokuts Indian. The book tells how Indians were recruited to the California Missions, how the Indians were treated in the California Missions and why Estanislao lead a revolution against the Mission system. Estanislao was a real person. He is a great American hero. Please see www.abeduspress.com for more information. We should teach our children the truth about the California Missions. The cost outside California is $11.99. The cost inside California is $12.65.